Mood Disorders

Mood Disorders

Editor: Sheila Reid

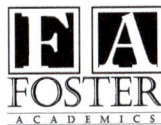

FA
FOSTER
ACADEMICS

www.fosteracademics.com

www.fosteracademics.com

FA
FOSTER
ACADEMICS

Cataloging-in-Publication Data

Mood disorders / edited by Sheila Reid.
   p. cm.
Includes bibliographical references and index.
ISBN 978-1-63242-557-7
1. Affective disorders. 2. Psychology, Pathological. I. Reid, Sheila.
RC537 .M66 2018
616.852 7--dc23

Foster Academics,
118-35 Queens Blvd., Suite 400,
Forest Hills, NY 11375, USA

ISBN 978-1-63242-557-7 (Hardback)

This book contains information obtained from authentic and highly regarded sources. All chapters are published with permission under the Creative Commons Attribution Share Alike License or equivalent. A wide variety of references are listed. Permissions and sources are indicated; for detailed attributions, please refer to the permissions page. Reasonable efforts have been made to publish reliable data and information, but the authors, editors and publisher cannot assume any responsibility for the vailidity of all materials or the consequences of their use.

Trademark Notice: Registered trademark of products or corporate names are used only for explanation and identification without intent to infringe.

Contents

Preface

A person's mental well-being is as important as a person's physical state. Mood disorders are the type of disorders which directly affect the mood of a person, making them deeply depressed, lonely or unusually happy in the span of few minutes. These disorders can be classified into cyclothymic disorder, bipolar disorder, dysthymic disorder, clinical depression, etc. This book attempts to understand the varied disorders that fall under the discipline of mood disorders and how such diseases affect in the daily life and cause physical problems in the lives of the patients. Most of the topics introduced in it cover new diagnostic and treatment techniques of mood disorders. This textbook will serve as a reference to a broad spectrum of readers.

A foreword of all chapters of the book is provided below:

Chapter 1 - An unwanted variation or change in an individual's mood, whose underlying clinical causes are a group of diseases are together termed as mood disorders. They are diagnosed by studying long-term mental states of an individual. This is an introductory chapter which will introduce briefly all the significant aspects of mood disorders; **Chapter 2 -** The various types of mood disorders, as popularly classified, include mania, hypomania, major depressive disorder and bipolar disorder. They cover the spectrum of a person's elevated and depressed mental states. This chapter has been carefully written to provide an easy understanding of the varied facets of mood disorders; **Chapter 3 -** Mood disorders can have severe, often crippling symptoms. Some of these which have been listed in this section include hallucination, emotional dysregulation, mood swing, depression and racing thoughts. The topics discussed in the chapter are of great importance to broaden the existing knowledge on mood disorders; **Chapter 4 -** Anxiety disorders are a group of mental disorders whose symptoms include anxiety and fear. Individuals often exhibit a variety of anxiety disorders and phobias at the same time. Mood disorders are best understood in confluence with the major topics listed in the following chapter; **Chapter 5 -** Cognitive behavioral therapy is a form of psychosocial treatment that helps in altering undesired thoughts and habits. It has been shown to be effective in treating milder forms of anxiety and depression disorders, substance abuse problems and posttraumatic stress disorder. The aspects elucidated in this chapter are of vital importance, and provide a better understanding of mood disorders.

At the end, I would like to thank all the people associated with this book devoting their precious time and providing their valuable contributions to this book. I would also like to express my gratitude to my fellow colleagues who encouraged me throughout the process.

Editor

An Introduction to Mood Disorder

An unwanted variation or change in an individual's mood, whose underlying clinical causes are a group of diseases are together termed as mood disorders. They are diagnosed by studying long-term mental states of an individual. This is an introductory chapter which will introduce briefly all the significant aspects of mood disorders.

Mood Disorder

Mood disorder is a group of diagnoses in the *Diagnostic and Statistical Manual of Mental Disorders* (DSM) classification system where a disturbance in the person's mood is hypothesized to be the main underlying feature. The classification is known as mood (affective) disorders in International Classification of Diseases (ICD).

English psychiatrist Henry Maudsley proposed an overarching category of *affective disorder*. The term was then replaced by *mood disorder*, as the latter term refers to the underlying or longitudinal emotional state, whereas the former refers to the external expression observed by others.

Mood disorders fall into the basic groups of elevated mood, such as mania or hypomania; depressed mood, of which the best-known and most researched is major depressive disorder (MDD) (commonly called clinical depression, unipolar depression, or major depression); and moods which cycle between mania and depression, known as bipolar disorder (BD) (formerly known as manic depression). There are several subtypes of depressive disorders or psychiatric syndromes featuring less severe symptoms such as dysthymic disorder (similar to but milder than MDD) and cyclothymic disorder (similar to but milder than BD). Mood disorders may also be substance-induced or occur in response to a medical condition.

Classification

Depressive Disorders

Major depressive disorder (MDD), commonly called major depression, unipolar depression, or clinical depression, wherein a person has one or more major depressive episodes. After a single episode, Major Depressive Disorder (single episode) would be diagnosed. After more than one episode, the diagnosis becomes Major Depressive

Disorder (Recurrent). Depression without periods of mania is sometimes referred to as *unipolar depression* because the mood remains at the bottom "pole" and does not climb to the higher, manic "pole" as in bipolar disorder.

Individuals with a major depressive episode or major depressive disorder are at increased risk for suicide. Seeking help and treatment from a health professional dramatically reduces the individual's risk for suicide. Studies have demonstrated that asking if a depressed friend or family member has thought of committing suicide is an effective way of identifying those at risk, and it does not "plant" the idea or increase an individual's risk for suicide in any way. Epidemiological studies carried out in Europe suggest that, at this moment, roughly 8.5 percent of the world's population are suffering from a depressive disorder. No age group seems to be exempt from depression, and studies have found that depression appears in infants as young as 6 months old who have been separated from their mothers.

Depressive disorder is frequent in primary care and general hospital practice but is often undetected. Unrecognized depressive disorder may slow recovery and worsen prognosis in physical illness, therefore it is important that all doctors be able to recognize the condition, treat the less severe cases, and identify those requiring specialist care.

Diagnosticians recognize several subtypes or course specifiers:

- *Atypical depression* (*AD*) is characterized by mood reactivity (paradoxical anhedonia) and positivity, significant weight gain or increased appetite ("comfort eating"), excessive sleep or somnolence (hypersomnia), a sensation of heaviness in limbs known as leaden paralysis, and significant social impairment as a consequence of hypersensitivity to perceived interpersonal rejection. Difficulties in measuring this subtype have led to questions of its validity and prevalence.

- *Melancholic depression* is characterized by a loss of pleasure (anhedonia) in most or all activities, a failure of reactivity to pleasurable stimuli, a quality of depressed mood more pronounced than that of grief or loss, a worsening of symptoms in the morning hours, early-morning waking, psychomotor retardation, excessive weight loss, or excessive guilt.

- *Psychotic major depression* (*PMD*), or simply psychotic depression, is the term for a major depressive episode, in particular of melancholic nature, wherein the patient experiences psychotic symptoms such as delusions or, less commonly, hallucinations. These are most commonly mood-congruent (content coincident with depressive themes).

- *Catatonic depression* is a rare and severe form of major depression involving disturbances of motor behavior and other symptoms. Here, the person is mute and almost stuporose, and either is immobile or exhibits purposeless or even bizarre movements. Catatonic symptoms can also occur in schizophrenia or a manic episode, or can be due to neuroleptic malignant syndrome.

- *Postpartum depression* (*PPD*) is listed as a course specifier in DSM-IV-TR; it refers to the intense, sustained and sometimes disabling depression experienced by women after giving birth. Postpartum depression, which affects 10–15% of women, typically sets in within three months of labor, and lasts as long as three months. It is quite common for women to experience a short-term feeling of tiredness and sadness in the first few weeks after giving birth; however, postpartum depression is different because it can cause significant hardship and impaired functioning at home, work, or school as well as, possibly, difficulty in relationships with family members, spouses, or friends, or even problems bonding with the newborn. In the treatment of postpartum major depressive disorders and other unipolar depressions in women who are breastfeeding, nortriptyline, paroxetine (Paxil), and sertraline (Zoloft) are in general considered to be the preferred medications. Women with personal or family histories of mood disorders are at particularly high risk of developing postpartum depression.

- *Seasonal affective disorder* (*SAD*), also known as "winter depression" or "winter blues", is a specifier. Some people have a seasonal pattern, with depressive episodes coming on in the autumn or winter, and resolving in spring. The diagnosis is made if at least two episodes have occurred in colder months with none at other times over a two-year period or longer. It is commonly hypothesised that people who live at higher latitudes tend to have less sunlight exposure in the winter and therefore experience higher rates of SAD, but the epidemiological support for this proposition is not strong (and latitude is not the only determinant of the amount of sunlight reaching the eyes in winter). SAD is also more prevalent in people who are younger and typically affects more females than males.

- *Dysthymia* is a condition related to unipolar depression, where the same physical and cognitive problems are evident, but they are not as severe and tend to last longer (usually at least 2 years). The treatment of dysthymia is largely the same as for major depression, including antidepressant medications and psychotherapy.

- *Double depression* can be defined as a fairly depressed mood (dysthymia) that lasts for at least two years and is punctuated by periods of major depression.

- *Depressive Disorder Not Otherwise Specified* (DD-NOS) is designated by the code *311* for depressive disorders that are impairing but do not fit any of the officially specified diagnoses. According to the DSM-IV, DD-NOS encompasses *"any depressive disorder that does not meet the criteria for a specific disorder."* It includes the research diagnoses of *recurrent brief depression*, and *minor depressive disorder* listed below.

- *Depressive personality disorder* (DPD) is a controversial psychiatric diagnosis that denotes a personality disorder with depressive features. Originally included in the DSM-II, depressive personality disorder was removed from the DSM-III and DSM-III-R. Recently, it has been reconsidered for reinstatement as a diagnosis. Depressive personality disorder is currently described in Appendix B in the DSM-IV-TR as worthy of further study.

- *Recurrent brief depression* (*RBD*), distinguished from major depressive disorder primarily by differences in duration. People with RBD have depressive episodes about once per month, with individual episodes lasting less than two weeks and typically less than 2–3 days. Diagnosis of RBD requires that the episodes occur over the span of at least one year and, in female patients, independently of the menstrual cycle. People with clinical depression can develop RBD, and vice versa, and both illnesses have similar risks.

- *Minor depressive disorder*, or simply minor depression, which refers to a depression that does not meet full criteria for major depression but in which at least two symptoms are present for two weeks.

Bipolar Disorders

Bipolar disorder (BD) (also called Manic Depression or Manic-Depressive Disorder), an unstable emotional condition characterized by cycles of abnormal, persistent high mood (mania) and low mood (depression), which was formerly known as "manic depression" (and in some cases rapid cycling, mixed states, and psychotic symptoms). Subtypes include:

- *Bipolar I* is distinguished by the presence or history of one or more manic episodes or mixed episodes with or without major depressive episodes. A depressive episode is not required for the diagnosis of Bipolar I Disorder, but depressive episodes are usually part of the course of the illness.

- *Bipolar II* consisting of recurrent intermittent hypomanic and depressive episodes or mixed episodes.

- *Cyclothymia* is a form of bipolar disorder, consisting of recurrent hypomanic and dysthymic episodes, but no full manic episodes or full major depressive episodes.

- *Bipolar Disorder Not Otherwise Specified* (*BD-NOS*), sometimes called "sub-threshold" bipolar, indicates that the patient suffers from some symptoms in the bipolar spectrum (e.g., manic and depressive symptoms) but does not fully qualify for any of the three formal bipolar DSM-IV diagnoses mentioned above.

It is estimated that roughly 1% of the adult population suffers from bipolar I, a further 1% suffers from bipolar II or cyclothymia, and somewhere between 2% and 5% percent suffer from "sub-threshold" forms of bipolar disorder. Furthermore the possibility of getting bipolar disorder when one parent is diagnosed with it is 15-30%. Risk when both parents have it is 50-75%. Also, while with bipolar siblings the risk is 15-25%, with identical twins it is about 70%.

A minority of people with bipolar disorder have high creativity, artistry or a particular gifted talent. Before the mania phase becomes too extreme, its energy, ambition, enthusiasm and grandiosity often bring people with this type of mood disorder life's masterpieces.

Substance-induced

A mood disorder can be classified as substance-induced if its etiology can be traced to the direct physiologic effects of a psychoactive drug or other chemical substance, or if the development of the mood disorder occurred contemporaneously with substance intoxication or withdrawal. Also, an individual may have a mood disorder coexisting with a substance abuse disorder. Substance-induced mood disorders can have features of a manic, hypomanic, mixed, or depressive episode. Most substances can induce a variety of mood disorders. For example, stimulants such as amphetamine, methamphetamine, and cocaine can cause manic, hypomanic, mixed, and depressive episodes.

Alcohol-induced

High rates of major depressive disorder occur in heavy drinkers and those with alcoholism. Controversy has previously surrounded whether those who abused alcohol and developed depression were self-medicating their pre-existing depression. But recent research has concluded that, while this may be true in some cases, alcohol misuse directly causes the development of depression in a significant number of heavy drinkers. Participants studied were also assessed during stressful events in their lives and measured on a *Feeling Bad Scale*. Likewise, they were also assessed on their affiliation with *deviant* peers, unemployment, and their partner's substance use and criminal offending. High rates of suicide also occur in those who have alcohol-related problems. It is usually possible to differentiate between alcohol-related depression and depression that is not related to alcohol intake by taking a careful history of the patient. Depression and other mental health problems associated with alcohol misuse may be due to distortion of brain chemistry, as they tend to improve on their own after a period of abstinence.

Benzodiazepine-induced

Benzodiazepines, such as alprazolam, clonazepam, lorazepam and diazepam, can cause both depression and mania.

Benzodiazepines are a class of medication commonly used to treat anxiety, panic attacks and insomnia, and are also commonly misused and abused. Those with anxiety, panic and sleep problems commonly have negative emotions and thoughts, depression, suicidal ideations, and often have comorbid depressive disorders. While the anxiolytic and hypnotic effects of benzodiazepines disappear as tolerance develops, depression and impulsivity with high suicidal risk commonly persist. Unfortunately, these symptoms are "often interpreted as an exacerbation or as a natural evolution of previous disorders and the chronic use of sedatives is overlooked." Benzodiazepines do not prevent the development of depression, can exacerbate preexisting depression, can cause depression in those with no history of it, and can lead to suicide attempts. Risk factors for attempted and completed suicide while using benzodiazepines include high dose prescriptions (even in those not misusing the medications), benzodiazepine intoxication, and underlying depression.

The long-term use of benzodiazepines may have a similar effect on the brain as alcohol, and are also implicated in depression. As with alcohol, the effects of benzodiazepine on neurochemistry, such as decreased levels of serotonin and norepinephrine, are believed to be responsible for the increased depression. Additionally, benzodiazepines can indirectly worsen mood by worsening sleep (i.e., benzodiazepine-induced sleep disorder). Like alcohol, benzodiazepines can put people to sleep but, while asleep, they disrupt sleep architecture: decreasing sleep time, delaying time to REM sleep, and decreasing deep sleep (the most restorative part of sleep for both energy and mood). Just as some antidepressants can cause or worsen anxiety in some patients due to being activating, benzodiazepines can cause or worsen depression due to being a central nervous system depressant—worsening thinking, concentration and problem solving (i.e., benzodiazepine-induced neurocognitive disorder). However, unlike antidepressants, in which the activating effects usually improve with continued treatment, benzodiazepine-induced depression is unlikely to improve until after stopping the medication.

In a long-term follow-up study of patients dependent on benzodiazepines, it was found that 10 people (20%) had taken drug overdoses while on chronic benzodiazepine medication despite only two people ever having had any pre-existing depressive disorder. A year after a gradual withdrawal program, no patients had taken any further overdoses.

Just as with intoxication and chronic use, benzodiazepine withdrawal can also cause depression. While benzodiazepine-induced depressive disorder may be exacerbated immediately after discontinuation of benzodiazepines, evidence suggests that mood significantly improves after the acute withdrawal period to levels better than during use. Depression resulting from withdrawal from benzodiazepines usually subsides after a few months but in some cases may persist for 6–12 months.

Due to Another Medical Condition

"Mood disorder due to a general medical condition" is used to describe manic or depressive episodes which occur secondary to a medical condition. There are many medical conditions that can trigger mood episodes, including neurological disorders (e.g. dementias), metabolic disorders (e.g. electrolyte disturbances), gastrointestinal diseases (e.g. cirrhosis), endocrine disease (e.g. thyroid abnormalities), cardiovascular disease (e.g. heart attack), pulmonary disease (e.g. chronic obstructive pulmonary disease), cancer, and autoimmune diseases (e.g. rheumatoid arthritis).

Not Otherwise Specified

Mood disorder not otherwise specified (MD-NOS) is a mood disorder that is impairing but does not fit in with any of the other officially specified diagnoses. In the DSM-IV MD-NOS is described as "any mood disorder that does not meet the criteria for a specific disorder." MD-NOS is not used as a clinical description but as a statistical concept for filing purposes.

Most cases of MD-NOS represent hybrids between mood and anxiety disorders, such as mixed anxiety-depressive disorder or atypical depression. An example of an instance of MD-NOS is being in minor depression frequently during various intervals, such as once every month or once in three days. There is a risk for MD-NOS not to get noticed, and for that reason not to get treated.

Cause

Meta-analyses show that high scores on the personality domain neuroticism is a strong predictor for the development of mood disorders. A number of authors have also suggested that mood disorders are an evolutionary adaptation. A low or depressed mood can increase an individual's ability to cope with situations in which the effort to pursue a major goal could result in danger, loss, or wasted effort. In such situations, low motivation may give an advantage by inhibiting certain actions. This theory helps to explain why negative life incidents precede depression in around 80 percent of cases, and why they so often strike people during their peak reproductive years. These characteristics would be difficult to understand if depression were a dysfunction.

A depressed mood is a predictable response to certain types of life occurrences, such as loss of status, divorce, or death of a child or spouse. These are events that signal a loss of reproductive ability or potential, or that did so in humans' ancestral environment. A depressed mood can be seen as an adaptive response, in the sense that it causes an individual to turn away from the earlier (and reproductively unsuccessful) modes of behavior.

A depressed mood is common during illnesses, such as influenza. It has been argued that this is an evolved mechanism that assists the individual in recovering by limiting his/her physical activity. The occurrence of low-level depression during the winter months, or seasonal affective disorder, may have been adaptive in the past, by limiting physical activity at times when food was scarce. It is argued that humans have retained the instinct to experience low mood during the winter months, even if the availability of food is no longer determined by the weather.

Much of what we know about the genetic influence of clinical depression is based upon research that has been done with identical twins. Identical twins both have exactly the same genetic code. It has been found that when one identical twin becomes depressed the other will also develop clinical depression approximately 76% of the time. When identical twins are raised apart from each other, they will both become depressed about 67% of the time. Because both twins become depressed at such a high rate, the implication is that there is a strong genetic influence. If it happened that when one twin becomes clinically depressed the other always develops depression, then clinical depression would likely be entirely genetic.

Diagnosis

DSM-5

The DSM-5, released in May 2013, separates the mood disorder chapter from the DSM-TR-IV into two sections: Depressive and Related Disorders and Bipolar and Related Disorders. Bipolar Disorders falls in between Depressive Disorders and Schizophrenia Spectrum and Related Disorders "in recognition of their place as a bridge between the two diagnostic classes in terms of symptomatology, family history and genetics" (Ref. 1, p 123). Bipolar Disorders underwent a few changes in the DSM-5, most notably the addition of more specific symptomology related to hypomanic and mixed manic states. Depressive Disorders underwent the most changes, the addition of three new disorders: disruptive mood dysregulation disorder, persistent depressive disorder (previously dysthymia), and premenstrual dysphoric disorder (previously in Appendix B, the section for disorders needing further research). Disruptive mood dysregulation disorder is meant as a diagnosis for children and adolescents who would normally be diagnosed with bipolar disorder as a way to limit the bipolar diagnosis in this age cohort. Major depressive disorder (MDD) also underwent a notable change, in that the bereavement clause has been removed. Those previously exempt from a diagnosis of MDD due to bereavement are now candidates for the MDD diagnosis.

Treatment

There are different types of treatments available for mood disorders, such as therapy and medications. Behaviour therapy, cognitive behaviour therapy and interpersonal therapy have all shown to be potentially beneficial in depression. Major depressive disorder medications usually include antidepressants, while bipolar disorder medications can consist of antipsychotics, mood stabilizers and/or lithium. Lithium specifically has been proven to reduce suicide and all causes of mortality in people with mood disorders.

Epidemiology

According to a substantial amount of epidemiology studies conducted, women are twice as likely to develop certain mood disorders, such as major depression. Although there is an equal number of men and women diagnosed with bipolar II disorder, women have a slightly higher frequency of the disorder.

In 2011, mood disorders were the most common reason for hospitalization among children aged 1–17 years in the United States, with approximately 112,000 stays. Mood disorders were top principal diagnosis for Medicaid super-utilizers in the United States in 2012. Further, a study of 18 States found that mood disorders accounted for the highest number of hospital readmissions among Medicaid patients and the uninsured, with 41,600 Medicaid patients and 12,200 uninsured patients being readmitted within 30 days of their index stay—a readmission rate of 19.8 per 100 admissions and 12.7 per 100 admissions, respectively. In 2012, mood and other behavioral health disorders were the most common diagnoses for Medicaid-covered and uninsured hospital stays in the United States (6.1% of Medicaid stays and 5.2% of uninsured stays).

A study conducted in 1988 to 1994 amongst young American adults involved a selection of demographic and health characteristics. A population-based sample of 8,602 men and women ages 17–39 years participated. Lifetime prevalence were estimated based on six mood measures:

1.   major depressive episode (MDE) 8.6%,

2.   major depressive disorder with severity (MDE-s) 7.7%,

3.   dysthymia 6.2%,

4.   MDE-s with dysthymia 3.4%,

5.   any bipolar disorder 1.6%, and

6.   any mood disorder 11.5%.

Research

Kay Redfield Jamison and others have explored the possible links between mood disorders — especially bipolar disorder — and creativity. It has been proposed that a "ruminating personality type may contribute to both [mood disorders] and art."

Jane Collingwood notes an Oregon State University study that

> "looked at the occupational status of a large group of typical patients and found that 'those with bipolar illness appear to be disproportionately concentrated in the most creative occupational category.' They also found that the likelihood of 'engaging in creative activities on the job' is significantly higher for bipolar than nonbipolar workers."

In Liz Paterek's article "Bipolar Disorder and the Creative Mind" she wrote

"Memory and creativity are related to mania. Clinical studies have shown that those in a manic state will rhyme, find synonyms, and use alliteration more than controls. This mental fluidity could contribute to an increase in creativity. Moreover, mania creates increases in productivity and energy. Those in a manic state are more emotionally sensitive and show less inhibition about attitudes, which could create greater expression. Studies performed at Harvard looked into the amount of original thinking in solving creative tasks. Bipolar individuals, whose disorder was not severe, tended to show greater degrees of creativity."

The relationship between depression and creativity appears to be especially strong among poets.

Mood (Psychology)

In psychology, a mood is an emotional state. In contrast to emotions, feelings, or affects, moods are less specific, less intense and less likely to be triggered by a particular stimulus or event. Moods are typically described as having either a positive or negative valence. In other words, people usually speak of being in a good mood or a bad mood.

Mood also differs from temperament or personality traits which are even longer-lasting. Nevertheless, personality traits such as optimism and neuroticism predispose certain types of moods. Long term disturbances of mood such as clinical depression and bipolar disorder are considered mood disorders. Mood is an internal, subjective state but it often can be inferred from posture and other behaviors. "We can be sent into a mood by an unexpected event, from the happiness of seeing an old friend to the anger of discovering betrayal by a partner. We may also just fall into a mood."

Research also shows that a person's mood can influence how they process advertising. Mood has been found to interact with gender to affect consumer processing of information.

Recent study separets 'mood' from 'emotions', as mood is the power of the mind and emotions are the traits of mind. As a powerhouse of mind 'mood' stimulates the activities of not only emotional faculties, but the faculties of memory, intelligence, and physical activities also. When the mood is degraded or depressed the activities of all the faculties are also diminished (Das K).

Etymology

Etymologically, the word *mood* derives from the Old English *mōd* which denoted military courage, but could also refer to a person's humor, temper, or disposition at a particular time. The cognate Gothic *mōds* translates both "mood, spiritedness" and "anger".

Types of Mood

Positive Mood

Positive mood can be caused by many different aspects of life as well as have certain effects on people as a whole. Good mood is usually considered a state without an identified cause; people cannot pinpoint exactly why they are in a good mood. People seem to experience a positive mood when they have a clean slate, have had a good night sleep, and feel no sense of stress in their life.

There have been many studies done on the effect of positive emotion on the cognitive mind and there is speculation that positive mood can affect our minds in good or bad ways. Generally, positive mood has been found to enhance creative problem solving and flexible yet careful thinking. Some studies have stated that positive moods let people think creatively, freely, and be more imaginative. Positive mood can also help individuals in situations in which heavy thinking and brainstorming is involved. In one experiment, individuals who were induced with a positive mood enhanced performance on the Remote Associates Task (RAT), a cognitive task that requires creative problem solving. Moreover, the study also suggests that being in a positive mood broadens or expands the breadth of attentional selection such that information that may be useful to the task at hand becomes more accessible for use. Consequently, greater accessibility of relevant information facilitates successful problem solving. Positive mood also facilitates resistance to temptations, especially with regards to unhealthy food choices.

Positive mood has also been proven to show negative effects on cognition as well. According to the article "Positive mood is associated with implicit use of distraction", "There is also evidence that individuals in positive moods show disrupted performance, at least when distracting information is present". The article states that other things in their peripheral views can easily distract people who are in good moods; an example of this would be if you were trying to study in the library (considering you are in a positive mood) you see people constantly walking around or making small noises. The study is basically stating that it would be harder for positive moods to focus on the task at hand. In particular, happy people may be more sensitive to the hedonic consequences of message processing than sad people. Thus, positive moods are predicted to lead to decreased processing only when thinking about the message is mood threatening. In comparison, if message processing allows a person to maintain or enhance a pleasant state then positive moods need not lead to lower levels of message scrutiny than negative moods. It is assumed that initial information regarding the source either confirms or disconfirms mood-congruent expectations. Specifically, a positive mood may lead to more positive expectations concerning source trustworthiness or likability than a negative mood. As a consequence, people in a positive mood should be more surprised when they encounter an untrustworthy or dislikable source rather than a trustworthy or likable source.

Negative Mood

Like positive moods, negative moods have important implications for human mental and physical wellbeing. Moods are basic psychological states that can occur as a reaction to an event or can surface for no apparent external cause. Since there is no intentional object that causes the negative mood, it has no specific start and stop date. It can last for hours, days, weeks, or longer. Negative moods can manipulate how individuals interpret and translate the world around them, and can also direct their behavior.

Negative moods can affect an individual's judgment and perception of objects and events. In a study done by Niedenthal and Setterlund (1994), research showed that individuals are tuned to perceive things that are congruent with their current mood. Negative moods, mostly low-intense, can control how humans perceive emotion-congruent objects and events. For example, Niedenthal and Setterland used music to induce positive and negative moods. Sad music was used as a stimulus to induce negative moods, and participants labeled other things as negative. This proves that people's current moods tend to affect their judgments and perceptions. These negative moods may lead to problems in social relationships. For example, one maladaptive negative mood regulation is an overactive strategy in which individuals over dramatize their negative feelings in order to provoke support and feedback from others and to guarantee their availability. A second type of maladaptive negative mood regulation is a disabling strategy in which individuals suppress their negative feelings and distance themselves from others in order to avoid frustrations and anxiety caused by others' unavailability.

Negative moods have been connected with depression, anxiety, aggression, poor self-esteem, physiological stress and decrease in sexual arousal. In some individuals, there is evidence that depressed or anxious mood may increase sexual interest or arousal. In general, men were more likely than women to report increased sexual drive during negative mood states. Negative moods are labeled as nonconstructive because it can affect a person's ability to process information; making them focus solely on the sender of a message, while people in positive moods will pay more attention to both the sender and the context of a message. This can lead to problems in social relationships with others.

Negative moods, such as anxiety, often lead individuals to misinterpret physical symptoms. According to Jerry Suls, a professor at the University of Iowa, people who are depressed and anxious tend to be in rumination. However, although an individual's affective states can influence the somatic changes, these individuals are not hypochondriacs.

Although negative moods are generally characterized as bad, not all negative moods are necessarily damaging. The Negative State Relief Model states that human beings have an innate drive to reduce negative moods. People can reduce their negative moods by engaging in any mood-elevating behavior (called Mood repair strategies), such as helping behavior, as it is paired with positive value such as smiles and thank you. Thus negative mood increases helpfulness because helping others can reduce one's own bad feelings.

Factors Which Affect Mood

Lack of Sleep

Sleep has a complex, and as of yet not fully elucidated, relationship with mood. Most commonly if a person is sleep deprived he/she will become more irritable, angry, more prone to stress, and less energized throughout the day. "Studies have shown that even partial sleep deprivation has a significant effect on mood. University of Pennsylvania researchers found that subjects who were limited to only 4.5 hours of sleep a night for one week reported feeling more stressed, angry, sad, and mentally exhausted. When the subjects resumed normal sleep, they reported a dramatic improvement in mood." Generally, evening oriented people, as compared to morning ones, show decreased energy and pleasantness and heightened tension.

However, in a subset of cases sleep deprivation can, paradoxically, lead to increased energy and alertness and enhanced mood. This effect is most marked in persons with an eveningeness type (so called night-owls) and people suffering from depression. For this reason it has, not surprisingly, been used as a treatment for major depressive disorder.

Nutrition

There is growing evidence that a diet rich in fruits and vegetables is related to greater happiness, life satisfaction, and positive mood. This evidence is independent of demographic or health variables including socio-economic status, exercise, smoking, and body mass index (BMI). Further studies have demonstrated a causal link between greater fruit and vegetable intake with feeling calmer, happier, more energetic, and more positive.

Facial Expression

Research studies have indicated that voluntary facial expressions, such as smiling, can produce effects on the body that are similar to those that result from the actual emotion, such as happiness. Paul Ekman and his colleagues have studied facial expressions of emotions and have linked specific emotions to the movement of specific facial muscles. Each basic emotion is associated with a distinctive facial expression. Sensory feedback from the expression contributes to the emotional feeling. Example: Smiling if you want to feel happy. Facial expressions have a large effect on self-reported anger and happiness which then affects your mood. Ekman has found that these expressions of emotion are universal and recognizable across widely divergent cultures.

Mood Disorders

Depression, chronic stress, bipolar disorder, etc. are considered mood disorders. It has been suggested that such disorders result from chemical imbalances in the brain's neurotransmitters, however some research challenges this hypothesis.

Social Mood

The idea of social mood as a "collectively shared state of mind" (Nofsinger 2005; Olson 2006) is attributed to Robert Prechter and his socionomics. The notion is used primarily in the field of economics (investments).

In sociology, philosophy, and psychology, crowd behavior is the formation of a *common mood* directed toward an object of attention.

References

- Lykins, A. D.; Janssen, E.; Graham, C. A. (2006). "The Relationship Between Negative Mood and Sexuality In Heterosexual College Women and Men". Journal of Sex Research. 43 (2): 136. doi:10.1080/00224490609552308

- Mezzich, Juan E. (2002). "International Surveys on the Use of ICD-10 and Related Diagnostic Systems" (guest editorial, abstract). Psychopathology. 35 (2–3): 72–75. PMID 12145487. doi:10.1159/000065122. Retrieved 2008-09-02

- Mayes, R.; Horwitz, AV. (2005). "DSM-III and the revolution in the classification of mental illness". J Hist Behav Sci. 41 (3): 249–67. PMID 15981242. doi:10.1002/jhbs.20103

- Lane, Christopher (2007). Shyness: How Normal Behavior Became a Sickness. Yale University Press. p. 263. ISBN 0-300-12446-5

- Sucală, M. L.; Tătar, A. (2010). "Optimism, pessimism and negative mood regulation expectancies in cancer patients". Journal of Cognitive and Behavioral Psychotherapies. 10 (1): 13–24

- Cassels, Caroline (2 December 2012). "DSM-5 Gets APA's Official Stamp of Approval". Medscape. WebMD, LLC. Retrieved 2012-12-05

- Kinderman, Peter (20 May 2013). "Explainer: what is the DSM?". The Conversation Australia. The Conversation Media Group. Retrieved 2013-05-21

- Niedenthal, P.M.; Setterlund, M.B. (1994). "Emotional congruence in perception". Personality and Social Psychology Bulletin. 20 (4): 401–411. doi:10.1177/0146167294204007

- Kendell, R.; Jablensky, A (January 2003). "Distinguishing Between the Validity and Utility of Psychiatric Diagnoses". American Journal of Psychiatry. 160 (1): 4–12. PMID 12505793. doi:10.1176/appi.ajp.160.1.4

- Catherine Pearson (20 May 2013). "DSM-5 Changes: What Parents Need To Know About The First Major Revision In Nearly 20 Years". The Huffington Post. Retrieved 2013-05-21

- Mayes, Rick; Bagwell, Catherine; Erkulwater, Jennifer L. (2009). "The Transformation of Mental Disorders in the 1980s: The DSM-III, Managed Care, and "Cosmetic Psychopharmacology"". Medicating Children: ADHD and Pediatric Mental Health. Harvard University Press. p. 76. ISBN 978-0-674-03163-0. Retrieved 2013-12-03

- Kress, Victoria (July 2014). "The Removal of the Multiaxial System in the DSM-5: Implications and Practice Suggestions for Counselors". The Professional Counselor Journal. 4 (3): 191–201

- Martin, E. A.; Kerns, J. G. (2011). "The influence of positive mood on different aspects of cognitive control". Cognition & Emotion. 25 (2): 265–279. doi:10.1080/02699931.2010.491652

- Zulu, Itibari M. "The Azibo Nosology: An Interview with Daudi Ajani ya Azibo" (PDF). Journal of Pan African Studies. 7 (5): 209–214

- Hands, D. Wade (December 2004). "On Operationalisms and Economics". Journal of Economic Issues. 38 (4): 953–968. doi:10.1080/00213624.2004.11506751

- Biss, R. K.; Hasher, L.; Thomas, R. C. (2010). "Positive mood is associated with the implicit use of distraction". Motivation & Emotion. 34 (1): 73–77. doi:10.1007/s11031-010-9156-y

- Atwell Irene; Azibo Daudi A (1991). "Diagnosing personality disorder in Africans (Blacks) using the Azibo nosology: Two case studies". Journal of Black Psychology. 17 (2): 1–22. doi:10.1177/00957984910172002

- Frances, Allen J. (December 2, 2012). "DSM 5 Is Guide Not Bible—Ignore Its Ten Worst Changes: APA approval of DSM-5 is a sad day for psychiatry". Psychology Today. Retrieved 2013-03-09

- Stuart A, Kirk; Herb Kutchins (1994). "The Myth of the Reliability of DSM". Journal of Mind and Behavior, 15(1&2). Archived from the original on 2008-03-07

- Spitzer, First (2005). "Classification of Psychiatric Disorders". JAMA. 294 (15): 1898–1899. doi:10.1001/jama.294.15.1898

2

Types of Mood Disorders

The various types of mood disorders, as popularly classified, include mania, hypomania, major depressive disorder and bipolar disorder. They cover the spectrum of a person's elevated and depressed mental states. This chapter has been carefully written to provide an easy understanding of the varied facets of mood disorders.

Mania

Mania is a state of abnormally elevated arousal, affect, and energy level, or "a state of heightened overall activation with enhanced affective expression together with lability of affect." Although mania is often conceived as a "mirror image" to depression, the heightened mood can be either euphoric or irritable; indeed, as the mania intensifies, irritability can be more pronounced and result in violence.

The nosology of the various stages of a manic episode has changed over the decades. The word derives from the Greek (*mania*), "madness, frenzy" and the verb (*mainomai*), "to be mad, to rage, to be furious".

The symptoms of mania are the following: heightened mood (either euphoric or irritable); flight of ideas and pressure of speech; and increased energy, decreased need for sleep, and hyperactivity. They are most plainly evident in fully developed hypomanic states; in full-blown mania, however, they undergo progressively severe exacerbations and become more and more obscured by other signs and symptoms, such as delusions and fragmentation of behavior.

Mania is a syndrome of multiple causes. Although the vast majority of cases occur in the context of bipolar disorder, it is a key component of other psychiatric disorders (as schizoaffective disorder, bipolar type) and may also occur secondary to various general medical conditions, as multiple sclerosis; certain medications, as prednisone; or certain substances of abuse, as cocaine or anabolic steroids. In current DSM-5 nomenclature, hypomanic episodes are separated from the more severe full manic episodes, which, in turn, are characterized as either mild, moderate, or severe, with specifiers with regard to certain symptomatic features (e.g. catatonia, psychosis). Mania, however, may be divided into three stages: hypomania, or stage I; acute mania, or stage II; and delirious mania, or stage III. This "staging" of a manic episode is, in particular, very useful from a descriptive and differential diagnostic point of view.

Mania varies in intensity, from mild mania (hypomania) to delirious mania, marked by such symptoms as disorientation, florid psychosis, incoherence, and catatonia. Standardized tools such as Altman Self-Rating Mania Scale and Young Mania Rating Scale can be used to measure severity of manic episodes. Because mania and hypomania have also long been associated with creativity and artistic talent, it is not always the case that the clearly manic bipolar person needs or wants medical help; such persons often either retain sufficient self-control to function normally or are unaware that they have "gone manic" severely enough to be committed or to commit themselves. Manic persons often can be mistaken for being on drugs.

Classification

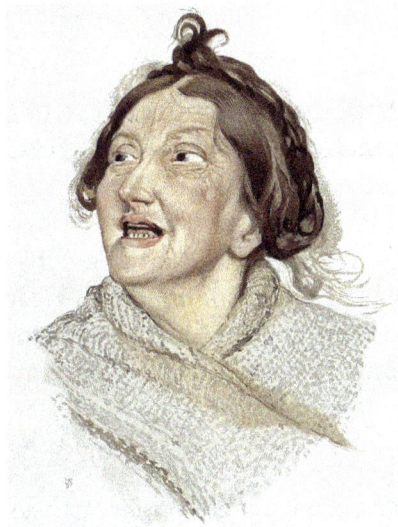

Lithograph from 1892 of a woman diagnosed with mania.

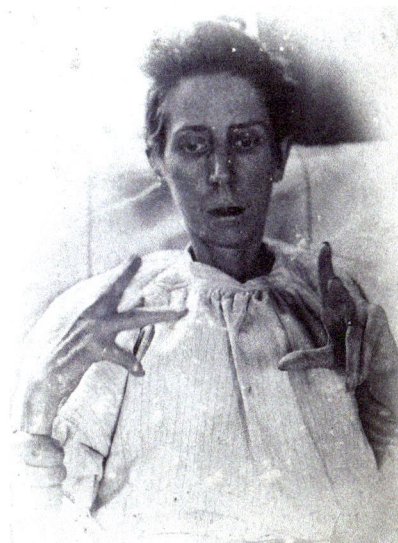

Friern Hospital, London; a woman with mania. Period 1890-1910

Mixed States

In a mixed affective state, the individual, though meeting the general criteria for a hypomanic (discussed below) or manic episode, experiences three or more concurrent depressive symptoms. This has caused some speculation, among clinicians, that mania and depression, rather than constituting "true" polar opposites, are, rather, two independent axes in a unipolar—bipolar spectrum.

A mixed affective state, especially with prominent manic symptoms, places the patient at a greater risk for completed suicide. Depression on its own is a risk factor but, when coupled with an increase in energy and goal-directed activity, the patient is far more likely to act with violence on suicidal impulses.

Hypomania

Hypomania is a lowered state of mania that does little to impair function or decrease quality of life. It may, in fact, increase productivity and creativity. In hypomania, there is less need for sleep and both goal-motivated behaviour and metabolism increase. Though the elevated mood and energy level typical of hypomania could be seen as a benefit, mania itself generally has many undesirable consequences including suicidal tendencies, and hypomania can, if the prominent mood is irritable rather than euphoric, be a rather unpleasant experience. By definition, hypomania cannot feature psychosis, nor can it require psychiatric hospitalisation (voluntary or involuntary).

Associated Disorders

A single manic episode, in the absence of secondary causes, (i.e., substance use disorder, pharmacologic, general medical condition) is sufficient to diagnose bipolar I disorder. Hypomania may be indicative of bipolar II disorder. Manic episodes are often complicated by delusions and/or hallucinations; should the psychotic features persist for a duration significantly longer than the episode of mania (two weeks or more), a diagnosis of schizoaffective disorder is more appropriate. Certain of "obsessive-compulsive spectrum" disorders as well as impulse control disorders share the name "mania," namely, kleptomania, pyromania, and trichotillomania. Despite the unfortunate association implied by the name, however, no connection exists between mania or bipolar disorder and these disorders. B_{12} deficiency can also cause characteristics of mania and psychosis.

Hyperthyroidism can produce similar symptoms to those of mania, such as agitation, elevated mood, increased energy, hyperactivity, sleep disturbances and sometimes, especially in severe cases, psychosis.

Signs and Symptoms

A manic episode is defined in the American Psychiatric Association's diagnostic manual as a "distinct period of abnormally and persistently elevated, expansive, or irritable mood and abnormally and persistently increased activity or energy, lasting at least 1 week and present most of the day, nearly every day (or any duration if hospitalization is necessary)," where the mood is not caused by drugs/medication or a medical illness (e.g., hyperthyroidism), and (a) is causing obvious difficulties at work or in social relationships and activities, or (b) requires admission to hospital to protect the person or others, or (c) the person is suffering psychosis.

To be classed as a manic episode, while the disturbed mood and an increase in goal directed activity or energy is present at least three (or four if only irritability is present) of the following must have been consistently present:

1. Inflated self-esteem or grandiosity

2. Decreased need for sleep (e.g., feels rested after 3 hours of sleep.)

3. More talkative than usual or pressure to keep talking.

4. Flights of ideas or subjective experience that thoughts are racing.

5. Increase in goal directed activity, or psychomotor acceleration.

6. Distractibility (too easily drawn to unimportant or irrelevant external stimuli).

7. Excessive involvement in activities with a high likelihood of painful consequences.(e.g., extravagant shopping, sexual adventures or improbable commercial schemes).

Though the activities one participates in while in a manic state are not *always* negative, those with the potential to have negative outcomes are far more likely.

If the person is concurrently depressed, they are said to be having a mixed episode.

The World Health Organization's classification system defines *a manic episode* as one where mood is higher than the person's situation warrants and may vary from relaxed high spirits to barely controllable exuberance, accompanied by hyperactivity, a compulsion to speak, a reduced sleep requirement, difficulty sustaining attention and often increased distractibility. Frequently, confidence and self-esteem are excessively enlarged, and grand, extravagant ideas are expressed. Behavior that is out of character and risky, foolish or inappropriate may result from a loss of normal social restraint.

Some people also have physical symptoms, such as sweating, pacing, and weight loss. In full-blown mania, often the manic person will feel as though his or her goal(s) trump all else, that there are no consequences or that negative consequences would be minimal, and that they need not exercise restraint in the pursuit of what they are after. Hypomania is different, as it may cause little or no impairment in function. The hypomanic person's connection with the external world, and its standards of interaction, remain intact, although intensity of moods is heightened. But those who suffer from prolonged unresolved hypomania do run the risk of developing full mania, and indeed may cross that "line" without even realizing they have done so.

One of the most signature symptoms of mania (and to a lesser extent, hypomania) is what many have described as racing thoughts. These are usually instances in which the manic person is excessively distracted by objectively unimportant stimuli. This experience creates an absent-mindedness where the manic individual's thoughts totally preoccupy him or her, making him or her unable to keep track of time, or be aware of anything besides the flow of thoughts. Racing thoughts also interfere with the ability to fall asleep.

Manic states are always relative to the normal state of intensity of the afflicted individual; thus, already irritable patients may find themselves losing their tempers even more quickly and an academically gifted person may, during the hypomanic stage, adopt seemingly "genius" characteristics and an ability to perform and articulate at a level far beyond that which would be capable during euthymia. A very simple indicator of a manic state would be if a heretofore clinically depressed patient suddenly becomes inordinately energetic, cheerful, aggressive, or "over happy." Other, often less obvious, elements of mania include delusions (generally of either grandeur or persecution, according to whether the predominant mood is euphoric or irritable), hypersensitivity, hyper vigilance, hypersexuality, hyper-religiosity, hyperactivity and impulsivity, a compulsion to over explain, (typically accompanied by pressure of speech) grandiose schemes and ideas, and a decreased need for sleep (for example, feeling rested after only 3 or 4 hours of sleep); in the case of the latter, the eyes of such patients may both look and feel abnormally "wide" or "open," rarely blinking, and this often contributing to some clinicians' erroneous belief that these patients are under the influence of a stimulant drug, when the patient, in fact, is either not on any mind-altering substances or is actually on a depressant drug, in a misguided attempt to ward off any undesirable manic symptoms. Individuals may also engage in out-of-character behavior during the episode, such as questionable business transactions, wasteful expenditures of money (e.g., spending sprees), risky sexual activity, abuse of recreational substances, excessive gambling, reckless behavior (as "speed driving" or daredevil activity), abnormal social interaction (as manifest via, for example, over familiarity and conversing with strangers), or highly vocal arguments. These behaviours may increase stress in personal relationships, lead to problems at work and increase the risk of altercations with law enforcement. There is a high risk of impulsively taking part in activities potentially harmful to self and others.

Although "severely elevated mood" sounds somewhat desirable and enjoyable, the experience of mania is ultimately often quite unpleasant and sometimes disturbing, if not frightening, for the person involved and for those close to them, and it may lead to impulsive behaviour that may later be regretted. It can also often be complicated by the sufferer's lack of judgment and insight regarding periods of exacerbation of characteristic states. Manic patients are frequently grandiose, obsessive, impulsive, irritable, belligerent, and frequently deny anything is wrong with them. Because mania frequently encourages high energy and decreased perception of need or ability to sleep, within a few days of a manic cycle, sleep-deprived psychosis may appear, further complicating the ability to think clearly. Racing thoughts and misperceptions lead to frustration and decreased ability to communicate with others.

Mania may also, as earlier mentioned, be divided into three "stages." Stage I corresponds with hypomania and may feature typical hypomanic characteristics, such as gregariousness and euphoria. In stages II and III mania, however, the patient may be extraordinarily irritable, psychotic or even delirious. These latter two stages are referred to as acute and delirious (or Bell's), respectively.

Cause

The biological mechanism by which mania occurs is not yet known. Based on the mechanism of action of antimanic agents (such as antipsychotics, valproate, tamoxifen, lithium, carbamazepine, etc.) and abnormalities seen in patients experiencing a manic episode the following is theorised to be involved in the pathophysiology of mania:

- Dopamine D2 receptor overactivity (which is a pharmacologic mechanism of antipsychotics in mania)

- GSK-3 overactivity

- Protein kinase C overactivity

- Inositol monophosphatase overactivity

- Increased arachidonic acid turnover

- Increased cytokine synthesis

Imaging studies have shown that the left amygdala is more active in women who are manic and the orbitofrontal cortex is less active. Pachygyria may be associated with mania also. During manic episodes decreased activity is found in the inferior frontal cortex.

Manic episodes may be triggered by dopamine receptor agonists, and this combined with increased VMAT2 activity support the role of dopamine in mania. Decreased cerebrospinal fluid levels of the serotonin metabolite 5-HIAA have been found in manic patients too, suggesting failure of serotonergic regulation and dopaminergic hyperactivity.

One proposed model for mania suggests that hyperactive fronto-striatal reward circuits result in manic symptoms.

Triggers

Various triggers have been associated with switching from euthymic or depressed states into mania. One common trigger of mania is antidepressant therapy. Studies show that the risk of switching while on an antidepressant is between 6-69% percent. Dopaminergic drugs such as reuptake inhibitors and dopamine agonists may also increase risk of switch. Other medication possibly include glutaminergic agents and drugs that alter the HPA axis. Lifestyle triggers include irregular sleep wake schedules and sleep deprivation, as well as extremely emotional or stressful stimuli.

Treatment

Before beginning treatment for mania, careful differential diagnosis must be performed to rule out secondary causes.

The acute treatment of a manic episode of bipolar disorder involves the utilization of either a mood stabilizer (valproate, lithium, or carbamazepine) or an atypical antipsychotic (olanzapine, quetiapine, risperidone, or aripiprazole). Although hypomanic episodes may respond to a mood stabilizer alone, full-blown episodes are treated with an atypical antipsychotic (often in conjunction with a mood stabilizer, as these tend to produce the most rapid improvement).

When the manic behaviours have gone, long-term treatment then focuses on prophylactic treatment to try to stabilize the patient's mood, typically through a combination of pharmacotherapy and psychotherapy. The likelihood of having a relapse is very high for those who have experienced two or more episodes of mania or depression. While medication for bipolar disorder is important to manage symptoms of mania and depression, studies show relying on medications alone is not the most effective method of treatment. Medication is most effective when used in combination with other bipolar disorder treatments, including psychotherapy, self-help coping strategies, and healthy lifestyle choices.

Lithium is the classic mood stabilizer to prevent further manic and depressive episodes. A systematic review found that long term lithium treatment substantially reduces the risk of bipolar manic relapse, by 42%. Anticonvulsants such as valproate, oxcarbazepine and carbamazepine are also used for prophylaxis. More recent drug solutions include lamotrigine, which is another anticonvulsant. Clonazepam (Klonopin) is also used. Sometimes atypical antipsychotics are used in combination with the previous mentioned medications as well, including olanzapine (Zyprexa) which helps treat hallucinations or delusions, Asenapine (Saphris, Sycrest), aripiprazole (Abilify), risperidone, ziprasidone, and clozapine which is often used for people who do not respond to lithium or anticonvulsants.

Verapamil, a calcium-channel blocker, is useful in the treatment of hypomania and in those cases where lithium and mood stabilizers are contraindicated or ineffective. Verapamil is effective for both short-term and long-term treatment.

Antidepressant monotherapy is not recommended for the treatment of depression in patients with bipolar disorders I or II, and no benefit has been demonstrated by combining antidepressants with mood stabilizers in these patients.

Society and Culture

In *Electroboy: A Memoir of Mania* by Andy Behrman, he describes his experience of mania as "the most perfect prescription glasses with which to see the world...life appears in front of you like an oversized movie screen". Behrman indicates early in his memoir that he sees himself not as a person suffering from an uncontrollable disabling illness, but as a director of the movie that is his vivid and emotionally alive life. "When I'm manic, I'm so awake and alert, that my eyelashes fluttering on the pillow sound like thunder". Many people who are artistic and do art in various forms have mania. Winston Churchill had periods of *manic symptoms* that may have been both an asset and a liability.

Hypomania

Hypomania (literally "under mania" or "less than mania") is a mood state characterized by persistent disinhibition and pervasive elevated (euphoric) with or without irritable mood but generally less severe than full mania. According to DSM-V criteria, hypomania is specifically distinct from mania in that there is no psychosis (sensing things others do not sense in the same environment); mania, by DSM-V definition, has psychotic features. Characteristic behaviors are extremely energetic, talkative, and confident commonly exhibited with a flight of creative ideas. While hypomanic behavior often generates productivity and excitement, it can become troublesome if the subject engages in risky or otherwise inadvisable behaviors. When manic episodes are "staged" according to symptomatic severity and associated features, hypomania constitutes the first stage, or stage I, of the syndrome, wherein the cardinal features (euphoria or heightened irritability, pressure of speech and activity, increased energy and decreased need for sleep, and flight of ideas) are most plainly evident.

Etymology

The Ancient Greek physician Hippocrates called one personality type 'hypomanic'. In 19th century psychiatry, when mania had a broad meaning of insanity, hypomania was equated by some to concepts of 'partial insanity' or monomania. A more specific usage was advanced by the German neuro-psychiatrist Emanuel Ernst Mendel in 1881, who wrote, "I recommend, taking into consideration the word used by Hippocrates, to name those types of mania that show a less severe phenomenological picture, 'hypomania'". Narrower operational definitions of hypomania were developed from the 1960s/1970s.

Signs and Symptoms

Individuals in a hypomanic state have a decreased need for sleep, are extremely outgoing and competitive, have a great deal of energy and are otherwise often fully functioning (unlike full mania).

Distinctive Markers

Specifically, hypomania is distinguished from mania by the absence of psychotic symptoms and grandiosity, and by its lesser degree of impact on functioning.

Hypomania is a feature of bipolar II disorder and cyclothymia, but can also occur in schizoaffective disorder. Hypomania is also a feature of bipolar I disorder as it arises in sequential procession as the mood disorder fluctuates between normal mood (euthymia) and mania. Some individuals with bipolar I disorder have hypomanic as well as manic episodes. Hypomania can also occur when moods progress downwards from a manic mood state to a normal mood. Hypomania is sometimes credited with increasing creativity and productive energy.

People who experience hyperthymia, or "chronic hypomania", encounter the same symptoms as hypomania but long-term.

Associated Disorders

Cyclothymia, a condition of continuous mood fluctuations, is characterized by oscillating experiences of hypomania and depression that fail to meet the diagnostic criteria for either manic or major depressive episodes. These periods are often interspersed with periods of relatively normal (euthymic) functioning.

When a patient presents with a history of at least one episode of both hypomania and major depression, each of which meet the diagnostic criteria, bipolar II disorder is diagnosed. In some cases, depressive episodes routinely occur during the fall or winter and hypomanic ones in the spring or early summer and, in such cases, one speaks of a "seasonal pattern".

If left untreated, and in those so predisposed, hypomania may transition into full-blown mania, which may be psychotic, in which case bipolar I disorder is the correct diagnosis.

Pathophysiology

Mania and hypomania are usually studied together in bipolar and the pathophysiology is usually assumed to be the same. Given that norepinephrine and dopaminergic drugs are capable of triggering hypomania, theories relating to monoamine hyperactivity have been proposed. A theory unifying depression and mania in bipolar proposes that decreased serotonergic regulation of other monoamines can result in either depressive or manic symptoms. Lesions on the right side frontal and temporal lobes have further been associated with mania.

Causes

Often in those who have experienced their first episode of hypomania – generally without psychotic features – there might be a long or recent history of depression or a mix of hypomania combined with depression known as mixed state prior to the emergence of manic symptoms, and commonly this surfaces in the mid to late teens. Due to this being an emotionally charged time, it is not unusual for mood swings to be passed off as hormonal or teenage ups and downs and for a diagnosis of bipolar disorder to be missed until there is evidence of an obvious manic/hypomanic phase.

Hypomania may also occur as a side effect of pharmaceuticals prescribed for conditions/diseases other than psychological states or mood disorders. In those instances, as in cases of drug-induced hypomanic episodes in unipolar depressives, the hypomania can almost invariably be eliminated by lowering medication dosage, withdrawing the drug entirely, or changing to a different medication if discontinuation of treatment is not possible.

Hypomania may also be triggered by the occurrence of a highly exciting event in the patient's situation, such as a substantial financial gain or recognition.

Hypomania can be associated with narcissistic personality disorder.

Evolution

Some commentators believe that hypomania actually has an evolutionary advantage. People with hypomania are generally perceived as being energetic, euphoric, visionary, overflowing with new ideas, and sometimes overconfident and very charismatic, yet— unlike those with full mania—are sufficiently capable of coherent thought and action to participate in everyday activities. Like mania, there seems to be a significant correlation between hypomania and creativity. A person in the state of hypomania might be immune to fear and doubt and have negligible social and sexual inhibition. People experiencing hypomania usually have a very strong sex drive. Hypomanic people are often the "life of the party". They may talk to strangers easily, offer solutions to problems, and find pleasure in small activities. Such advantages may render them unwilling to submit to treatment, especially when symptoms do not impair functioning.

Diagnosis

The DSM-IV-TR defines a hypomanic episode as including, over the course of at least four days, elevated mood plus three of the following symptoms OR irritable mood plus four of the following symptoms:

- pressured speech
- inflated self-esteem or grandiosity
- decreased need for sleep
- flight of ideas or the subjective experience that thoughts are racing

- easily distracted and attention-deficit similar to attention deficit hyperactivity disorder

- increase in psychomotor agitation

- hypersexuality

- involvement in pleasurable activities that may have a high potential for negative psycho-social or physical consequences (e.g., the person engages in unrestrained buying sprees, sexual indiscretions, reckless driving, or foolish business investments).

Treatment

Medications typically prescribed for hypomania include mood stabilizers such as valproic acid and lithium carbonate as well as atypical antipsychotics such as olanzapine and quetiapine. Putting someone with bipolar disorder on antidepressants can be hazardous as this may actually trigger more manic or hypomanic episodes.

If a hypomanic state is the result of medication side effects or drug abuse (e.g. amphetamines), then certain sedatives including benzodiazepines can sometimes normalize an individual's mood and energy levels.

Major Depressive Disorder

Major depressive disorder (MDD), also known simply as depression, is a mental disorder characterized by at least two weeks of low mood that is present across most situations. It is often accompanied by low self-esteem, loss of interest in normally enjoyable activities, low energy, and pain without a clear cause. People may also occasionally have false beliefs or see or hear things that others cannot. Some people have periods of depression separated by years in which they are normal while others nearly always have symptoms present. Major depressive disorder can negatively affect a person's personal, work, or school life, as well as sleeping, eating habits, and general health. Between 2–7% of adults with major depression die by suicide, and up to 60% of people who die by suicide had depression or another mood disorder.

The cause is believed to be a combination of genetic, environmental, and psychological factors. Risk factors include a family history of the condition, major life changes, certain medications, chronic health problems, and substance abuse. About 40% of the risk appears to be related to genetics. The diagnosis of major depressive disorder is based on the person's reported experiences and a mental status examination. There is no laboratory test for major depression. Testing, however, may be done to rule out physical conditions that can cause similar symptoms. Major depression should be differentiated from sadness which is a normal part of life and is less severe. The United States Preventive Services Task Force (USPSTF) recommends screening for depression among those over the age 12, while a prior Cochrane review found that the routine use of screening questionnaires have little effect on detection or treatment.

Typically, people are treated with counseling and antidepressant medication. Medication appears to be effective, but the effect may only be significant in the most severely depressed. It is unclear whether medications affect the risk of suicide. Types of counseling used include cognitive behavioral therapy (CBT) and interpersonal therapy. If other measures are not effective electroconvulsive therapy (ECT) may be tried. Hospitalization may be necessary in cases with a risk of harm to self and may occasionally occur against a person's wishes.

Major depressive disorder affected approximately 216 million people (3% of the world's population) in 2015. The percentage of people who are affected at one point in their life varies from 7% in Japan to 21% in France. Lifetime rates are higher in the developed world (15%) compared to the developing world (11%). It causes the second most years lived with disability after low back pain. The most common time of onset is in a person in their 20s and 30s. Females are affected about twice as often as males. The American Psychiatric Association added "major depressive disorder" to the *Diagnostic and Statistical Manual of Mental Disorders* (DSM-III) in 1980. It was a split of the previous depressive neurosis in the DSM-II which also encompassed the conditions now known as dysthymia and adjustment disorder with depressed mood. Those currently or previously affected may be stigmatized.

Signs and Symptoms

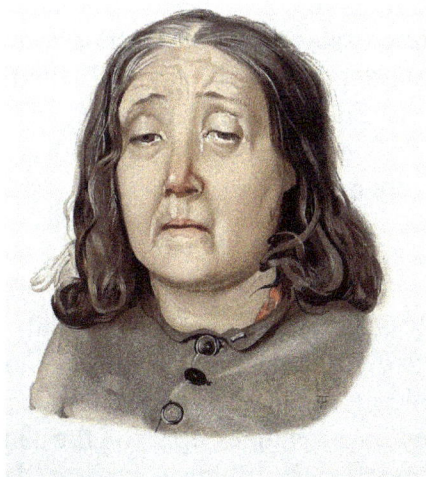

An 1892 lithograph of a woman diagnosed with depression

Major depression significantly affects a person's family and personal relationships, work or school life, sleeping and eating habits, and general health. Its impact on functioning and well-being has been compared to that of other chronic medical conditions such as diabetes.

A person having a major depressive episode usually exhibits a very low mood, which pervades all aspects of life, and an inability to experience pleasure in activities that were formerly enjoyed. Depressed people may be preoccupied with, or ruminate over, thoughts and feelings of worthlessness, inappropriate guilt or regret, helplessness, hopelessness, and self-hatred. In severe cases, depressed people may have symptoms of psychosis. These symptoms include delusions or, less commonly, hallucinations, usually unpleasant. Other symptoms of depression include poor concentration and memory (especially in those with melancholic or psychotic features), withdrawal from social situations and activities, reduced sex drive, irritability, and thoughts of death or suicide. Insomnia is common among the depressed. In the typical pattern, a person wakes very early and cannot get back to sleep. Hypersomnia, or oversleeping, can also happen. Some antidepressants may also cause insomnia due to their stimulating effect.

A depressed person may report multiple physical symptoms such as fatigue, headaches, or digestive problems; physical complaints are the most common presenting problem in developing countries, according to the World Health Organization's criteria for depression. Appetite often decreases, with resulting weight loss, although increased appetite and weight gain occasionally occur. Family and friends may notice that the person's behavior is either agitated or lethargic. Older depressed people may have cognitive symptoms of recent onset, such as forgetfulness, and a more noticeable slowing of movements. Depression often coexists with physical disorders common among the elderly, such as stroke, other cardiovascular diseases, Parkinson's disease, and chronic obstructive pulmonary disease.

Depressed children may often display an irritable mood rather than a depressed mood, and show varying symptoms depending on age and situation. Most lose interest in school and show a decline in academic performance. They may be described as clingy, demanding, dependent, or insecure. Diagnosis may be delayed or missed when symptoms are interpreted as normal moodiness.

Associated Conditions

Major depression frequently co-occurs with other psychiatric problems. The 1990–92 *National Comorbidity Survey* (US) reports that half of those with major depression also have lifetime anxiety and its associated disorders such as generalized anxiety disorder. Anxiety symptoms can have a major impact on the course of a depressive illness, with delayed recovery, increased risk of relapse, greater disability and increased suicide attempts. There are increased rates of alcohol and drug abuse and particularly dependence, and around a third of individuals diagnosed with ADHD develop comorbid depression. Post-traumatic stress disorder and depression often co-occur. Depression may also coexist with attention deficit hyperactivity disorder (ADHD), complicating the diagnosis and treatment of both. Depression is also frequently comorbid with alcohol abuse and personality disorders.

Depression and pain often co-occur. One or more pain symptoms are present in 65% of depressed patients, and anywhere from 5 to 85% of patients with pain will be suffering from depression, depending on the setting; there is a lower prevalence in general practice, and higher in specialty clinics. The diagnosis of depression is often delayed or missed, and the outcome worsens. The outcome can also worsen if the depression is noticed but completely misunderstood.

Depression is also associated with a 1.5- to 2-fold increased risk of cardiovascular disease, independent of other known risk factors, and is itself linked directly or indirectly to risk factors such as smoking and obesity. People with major depression are less likely to follow medical recommendations for treating and preventing cardiovascular disorders, which further increases their risk of medical complications. In addition, cardiologists may not recognize underlying depression that complicates a cardiovascular problem under their care.

Cause

The cause of major depressive disorder is unknown. The biopsychosocial model proposes that biological, psychological, and social factors all play a role in causing depression. The diathesis–stress model specifies that depression results when a preexisting vulnerability, or diathesis, is activated by stressful life events. The preexisting vulnerability can be either genetic, implying an interaction between nature and nurture, or schematic, resulting from views of the world learned in childhood.

Childhood abuse, either physical, sexual or psychological are all risk factors for depression, among other psychiatric issues that co-occur such as anxiety and drug abuse. Childhood trauma also correlates with severity of depression, lack of response to treatment and length of illness. However, some are more susceptible to developing mental illness such as depression after trauma, and various genes have been suggested to control susceptibility.

Genetics

The 5-HTTLPR, or serotonin transporter promoter gene's short allele has been associated with increased risk of depression. However, since the 1990s results have been inconsistent, with three recent reviews finding an effect and two finding none. Other genes that have been linked to a GxE interaction include CRHR1, FKBP5 and BDNF, the first two of which are related to the stress reaction of the HPA axis, and the latter of which is involved in neurogenesis.

Other Health Problems

Depression may also come secondary to a chronic or terminal medical conditioned such as HIV/AIDS, or asthma and may be labeled "secondary depression". It is unknown if the underlying diseases induce depression through effect on quality of life, of through shared etiologies (such as degeneration of the basal ganglia in parkinson's disease or immune dysregulation in asthma). Depression may also be iatrogenic (the result of healthcare), such as drug induced depression. Therapies associated with depression include interferon therapy, beta-blockers, Isotretinoin, contraceptives, cardiac agents, anticonvulsants, antimigraine drugs, antipsychotics, and hormonal agents agents such as gonadotropin-releasing hormone agonist. Drug abuse in early age is also associated with increased risk of developing depression later in life. Depression that occurs as a result of pregnancy is called postpartum depression, and is though to be the result of hormonal changes associated with pregnancy. Seasonal affective disorder, a type of depression associated with seasonal changes in sunlight, is though to be the result of decreased sunlight.

Pathophysiology

The pathophysiology of depression is not yet understood, but the current theories center around monoaminergic systems, the circadian rhythm, immunological dysfunction, HPA axis dysfunction and structural or functional abnormalities of emotional circuits.

The monoamine theory, derived from the efficacy of monoaminergic drugs in treating depression, was the dominant theory until recently. The theory postulates that insufficient activity of monoamine neurotransmitters is the primary cause of depression. Evidence for the monoamine theory comes from multiple areas. Firstly, acute depletion of tryptophan, a necessary precursor of serotonin, a monoamine, can cause depression in those in remission or relatives of depressed patients; this suggests that decreased serotonergic neurotransmission is important in depression. Secondly, the correlation between depression risk and polymorphisms in the 5-HTTLPR gene, which codes for serotonin receptors, suggests a link. Third, decreased size of the locus coeruleus, decreased activity of tyrosine hydroxylase, increased density of alpha-2 adrenergic receptor, and evidence from rat models suggest decreased adrenergic neurotransmission in depression. Furthermore, decreased levels of homovanillic acid, altered response to dextroamphetamine, responses of depressive symptoms to dopamine receptor agonists, decreased dopamine receptor D1 binding in the striatum, and polymorphism of dopamine receptor genes implicate dopamine in depression. Lastly, increased activity of monoamine oxidase, which degrades monoamines, has been associated with depression. However, this theory is inconsistent with the fact that serotonin depletion does not cause depression in healthy persons, the fact that antidepressants instantly increase levels of monoamines but take weeks to work, and the existence of atypical antidepressants which can be effective despite not targeting this pathway. One proposed explanation for the therapeutic lag, and further support for the deficiency of monoamines, is a desensitization of self-inhibition in raphe nuclei by the increased serotonin mediated by antidepressants. However, disinhibition of the dorsal raphe has been proposed to occur as a result of *decreased* serotonergic activity in tryptophan depletion, resulting in a depressed state mediated by increased serotonin. Further countering the monoamine hypothesis is the fact that rats with lesions of the dorsal raphe are not more depressive that controls, the finding of increased jugular 5-HIAA in depressed patients that normalized with SSRI treatment, and the preference for carbohydrates in depressed patients. Already limited, the monoamine hypothesis has been further oversimplified when presented to the general public.

Immune system abnormalities have been observed, including increased levels of cytokines involved in generating sickness behavior (which shares overlap with depression). The effectiveness of nonsteroidal anti-inflammatory drugs (NSAIDs) and cytokine inhibitors in treating depression, and normalization of cytokine levels after successful treatment further suggest immune system abnormalities in depression.

HPA axis abnormalities have been suggested in depression given the association of CRHR1 with depression and the increased frequency of dexamethasone test non-suppression in depressed patients. However, this abnormality is not adequate as a diagnosis tool, because its sensitivity is only 44%. These stress-related abnormalities have been hypothesized to be the cause of hippocampal volume reductions seen in depressed patients. Furthermore, a meta-analysis yielded decreased dexamethasone suppression, and increased response to psychological stressors. Further abnormal results have been obscured with the cortisol awakening response, with increased response being associated with depression.

Theories unifying neuroimaging findings have been proposed. The first model proposed is the "Limbic Cortical Model", which involves hyperactivity of the ventral paralimbic regions and hypoactivity of frontal regulatory regions in emotional processing. Another model, the "Corito-Striatal model", suggests that abnormalities of the prefrontal cortex in regulating striatal and subcortical structures results in depression. Another model proposes hyperactivity of salience structures in identifying negative stimuli, and hypoactivity of cortical regulatory structures resulting in a negative emotional bias and depression, consistent with emotional bias studies.

Diagnosis

Clinical Assessment

A diagnostic assessment may be conducted by a suitably trained general practitioner, or by a psychiatrist or psychologist, who records the person's current circumstances, biographical history, current symptoms, and family history. The broad clinical aim is to formulate the relevant biological, psychological, and social factors that may be impacting on the individual's mood. The assessor may also discuss the person's current ways of regulating mood (healthy or otherwise) such as alcohol and drug use. The assessment also includes a mental state examination, which is an assessment of the person's current mood and thought content, in particular the presence of themes of hopelessness or pessimism, self-harm or suicide, and an absence of positive thoughts or plans. Specialist mental health services are rare in rural areas, and thus diagnosis and management is left largely to primary-care clinicians. This issue is even more marked in developing countries. The mental health examination may include the use of a rating scale such as the Hamilton Rating Scale for Depression or the Beck Depression Inventory or the Suicide Behaviors Questionnaire-Revised. The score on a rating scale alone is insufficient to diagnose depression to the satisfaction of the DSM or ICD, but it provides an indication of the severity of symptoms for a time period, so a person who scores above a given cut-off point can be more thoroughly evaluated for a depressive disorder diagnosis. Several rating scales are used for this purpose.

Primary-care physicians and other non-psychiatrist physicians have more difficulty with underrecognition and undertreatment of depression compared to psychiatric physicians, in part because of the physical symptoms that often accompany depression, in addition to the many potential patient, provider, and system barriers that the authors describe. A review found that non-psychiatrist physicians miss about two-thirds of cases, though this has improved somewhat in more recent studies.

Before diagnosing a major depressive disorder, in general a doctor performs a medical examination and selected investigations to rule out other causes of symptoms. These include blood tests measuring TSH and thyroxine to exclude hypothyroidism; basic electrolytes and serum calcium to rule out a metabolic disturbance; and a full blood count including ESR to rule out a systemic infection or chronic disease. Adverse affective reactions to medications or alcohol misuse are often ruled out, as well. Testosterone levels may be evaluated to diagnose hypogonadism, a cause of depression in men. Vitamin D levels might be evaluated, as low levels of vitamin D have been associated with greater risk for depression.

Subjective cognitive complaints appear in older depressed people, but they can also be indicative of the onset of a dementing disorder, such as Alzheimer's disease. Cognitive testing and brain imaging can help distinguish depression from dementia. A CT scan can exclude brain pathology in those with psychotic, rapid-onset or otherwise unusual symptoms. In general, investigations are not repeated for a subsequent episode unless there is a medical indication.

No biological tests confirm major depression. Biomarkers of depression have been sought to provide an objective method of diagnosis. There are several potential biomarkers, including Brain-Derived Neurotrophic Factor and various functional MRI techniques. One study developed a decision tree model of interpreting a series of fMRI scans taken during various activities. In their subjects, the authors of that study were able to achieve a sensitivity of 80% and a specificity of 87%, corresponding to a negative predictive value of 98% and a positive predictive value of 32% (positive and negative likelihood ratios were 6.15, 0.23, respectively). However, much more research is needed before these tests could be used clinically.

DSM-IV-TR and ICD-10 Criteria

The most widely used criteria for diagnosing depressive conditions are found in the American Psychiatric Association's revised fourth edition of the *Diagnostic and Statistical Manual of Mental Disorders* (DSM-IV-TR), and the World Health Organization's *International Statistical Classification of Diseases and Related Health Problems* (ICD-10), which uses the name *depressive episode* for a single episode and *recurrent depressive disorder* for repeated episodes. The latter system is typically used in European countries, while the former is used in the US and many other non-European nations, and the authors of both have worked towards conforming one with the other.

Both DSM-IV-TR and ICD-10 mark out typical (main) depressive symptoms. ICD-10 defines three typical depressive symptoms (depressed mood, anhedonia, and reduced energy), two of which should be present to determine depressive disorder diagnosis. According to DSM-IV-TR, there are two main depressive symptoms—depressed mood and anhedonia. At least one of these must be present to make a diagnosis of major depressive episode.

Major depressive disorder is classified as a mood disorder in DSM-IV-TR. The diagnosis hinges on the presence of single or recurrent major depressive episodes. Further qualifiers are used to classify both the episode itself and the course of the disorder. The category Depressive Disorder Not Otherwise Specified is diagnosed if the depressive episode's manifestation does not meet the criteria for a major depressive episode. The ICD-10 system does not use the term *major depressive disorder* but lists very similar criteria for the diagnosis of a depressive episode (mild, moderate or severe); the term *recurrent* may be added if there have been multiple episodes without mania.

Major Depressive Episode

A major depressive episode is characterized by the presence of a severely depressed mood that persists for at least two weeks. Episodes may be isolated or recurrent and are categorized as mild (few symptoms in excess of minimum criteria), moderate, or severe (marked impact on social or occupational functioning). An episode with psychotic features—commonly referred to as *psychotic depression*—is automatically rated as severe. If the patient has had an episode of mania or markedly elevated mood, a diagnosis of bipolar disorder is made instead. Depression without mania is sometimes referred to as *unipolar* because the mood remains at one emotional state or "pole".

DSM-IV-TR excludes cases where the symptoms are a result of bereavement, although it is possible for normal bereavement to evolve into a depressive episode if the mood persists and the characteristic features of a major depressive episode develop. The criteria have been criticized because they do not take into account any other aspects of the personal and social context in which depression can occur. In addition, some studies have found little empirical support for the DSM-IV cut-off criteria, indicating they are a diagnostic convention imposed on a continuum of depressive symptoms of varying severity and duration: Excluded are a range of related diagnoses, including dysthymia, which involves a chronic but milder mood disturbance; recurrent brief depression, consisting of briefer depressive episodes; minor depressive disorder, whereby only some symptoms of major depression are present; and adjustment disorder with depressed mood, which denotes low mood resulting from a psychological response to an identifiable event or stressor.

Subtypes

The DSM-IV-TR recognizes five further subtypes of MDD, called *specifiers*, in addition to noting the length, severity and presence of psychotic features:

- Melancholic depression is characterized by a loss of pleasure in most or all activities, a failure of reactivity to pleasurable stimuli, a quality of depressed mood more pronounced than that of grief or loss, a worsening of symptoms in the morning hours, early-morning waking, psychomotor retardation, excessive weight loss, or excessive guilt.

- Atypical depression is characterized by mood reactivity (paradoxical anhedonia) and positivity, significant weight gain or increased appetite (comfort eating), excessive sleep or sleepiness (hypersomnia), a sensation of heaviness in limbs known as leaden paralysis, and significant social impairment as a consequence of hypersensitivity to perceived interpersonal rejection.

- Catatonic depression is a rare and severe form of major depression involving disturbances of motor behavior and other symptoms. Here, the person is mute and almost stuporous, and either remains immobile or exhibits purposeless or even bizarre movements. Catatonic symptoms also occur in schizophrenia or in manic episodes, or may be caused by neuroleptic malignant syndrome.

- Postpartum depression, or mental and behavioral disorders associated with the puerperium, not elsewhere classified, refers to the intense, sustained and sometimes disabling depression experienced by women after giving birth. Postpartum depression has an incidence rate of 10–15% among new mothers. The DSM-IV mandates that, in order to qualify as postpartum depression, onset occur within one month of delivery. It has been said that postpartum depression can last as long as three months.

- Seasonal affective disorder (SAD) is a form of depression in which depressive episodes come on in the autumn or winter, and resolve in spring. The diagnosis is made if at least two episodes have occurred in colder months with none at other times, over a two-year period or longer.

Screening

In 2016, the United States Preventive Services Task Force (USPSTF) recommended screening in the adult populations with evidence that it increases the detection of people with depression and with proper treatment improves outcomes. They recommend screening in those between the age of 12 to 18 as well.

A Cochrane review from 2005 found screening programs do not significantly improve detection rates, treatment, or outcome.

Differential Diagnoses

To confer major depressive disorder as the most likely diagnosis, other potential diagnoses must be considered, including dysthymia, adjustment disorder with depressed mood, or bipolar disorder. Dysthymia is a chronic, milder mood disturbance in which a person reports a low mood almost daily over a span of at least two years. The symptoms are not as severe as those for major depression, although people with dysthymia are vulnerable to secondary episodes of major depression (sometimes referred to as *double depression*). Adjustment disorder with depressed mood is a mood disturbance appearing as a psychological response to an identifiable event or stressor, in which the resulting emotional or behavioral symptoms are significant but do not meet the criteria for a major depressive episode. Bipolar disorder, also known as *manic–depressive disorder*, is a condition in which depressive phases alternate with periods of mania or hypomania. Although depression is currently categorized as a separate disorder, there is ongoing debate because individuals diagnosed with major depression often experience some hypomanic symptoms, indicating a mood disorder continuum. Further differential diagnoses involve chronic fatigue syndrome.

Other disorders need to be ruled out before diagnosing major depressive disorder. They include depressions due to physical illness, medications, and substance abuse. Depression due to physical illness is diagnosed as a Mood disorder due to a general medical condition. This condition is determined based on history, laboratory findings, or physical examination. When the depression is caused by a medication, drug of abuse, or exposure to a toxin, it is then diagnosed as a specific mood disorder (previously called *Substance-induced mood disorder* in the DSM-IV-TR).

Prevention

Preventative efforts may result in decreases in rates of the condition of between 22 and 38%. Eating large amounts of fish may also reduce the risk.

Behavioral interventions, such as interpersonal therapy and cognitive-behavioral therapy, are effective at preventing new onset depression. Because such interventions appear to be most effective when delivered to individuals or small groups, it has been suggested that they may be able to reach their large target audience most efficiently through the Internet.

However, an earlier meta-analysis found preventive programs with a competence-enhancing component to be superior to behavior-oriented programs overall, and found behavioral programs to be particularly unhelpful for older people, for whom social support programs were uniquely beneficial. In addition, the programs that best prevented depression comprised more than eight sessions, each lasting between 60 and 90 minutes, were provided by a combination of lay and professional workers, had a high-quality research design, reported attrition rates, and had a well-defined intervention.

The Netherlands mental health care system provides preventive interventions, such as the "Coping with Depression" course (CWD) for people with sub-threshold depression. The course is claimed to be the most successful of psychoeducational interventions for the treatment and prevention of depression (both for its adaptability to various populations and its results), with a risk reduction of 38% in major depression and an efficacy as a treatment comparing favorably to other psychotherapies.

Management

The three most common treatments for depression are psychotherapy, medication, and electroconvulsive therapy. Psychotherapy is the treatment of choice (over medication) for people under 18. The UK National Institute for Health and Care Excellence (NICE) 2004 guidelines indicate that antidepressants should not be used for the initial treatment of mild depression, because the risk-benefit ratio is poor. The guidelines recommend that antidepressants treatment in combination with psychosocial interventions should be considered for:

- People with a history of moderate or severe depression

- Those with mild depression that has been present for a long period

- As a second line treatment for mild depression that persists after other interventions

- As a first line treatment for moderate or severe depression.

The guidelines further note that antidepressant treatment should be continued for at least six months to reduce the risk of relapse, and that SSRIs are better tolerated than tricyclic antidepressants.

American Psychiatric Association treatment guidelines recommend that initial treatment should be individually tailored based on factors including severity of symptoms, co-existing disorders, prior treatment experience, and patient preference. Options may include pharmacotherapy, psychotherapy, exercise, electroconvulsive therapy (ECT), transcranial magnetic stimulation (TMS) or light therapy. Antidepressant medication is recommended as an initial treatment choice in people with mild, moderate, or severe major depression, and should be given to all patients with severe depression unless ECT is planned.

Treatment options are much more limited in developing countries, where access to mental health staff, medication, and psychotherapy is often difficult. Development of mental health services is minimal in many countries; depression is viewed as a phenomenon of the developed world despite evidence to the contrary, and not as an inherently life-threatening condition. A 2014 Cochrane review found insufficient evidence to determine the effectiveness of psychological versus medical therapy in children.

Lifestyle

Physical exercise is recommended for management of mild depression, and has a moderate effect on symptoms. Exercise has also been found to be effective for (unipolar) major depression. It is equivalent to the use of medications or psychological therapies in most people. In the older people it does appear to decrease depression. Exercise may be recommended to people who are willing, motivated, and physically healthy enough to participate in an exercise program as treatment.

There is a small amount of evidence that skipping a night's sleep may improve depressive symptoms, with the effects usually showing up within a day. This effect is usually temporary. Besides sleepiness, this method can cause a side effect of mania or hypomania.

In observational studies smoking cessation has benefits in depression as large as or larger than those of medications.

Besides exercise, sleep and diet may play a role in depression, and interventions in these areas may be an effective add on to conventional methods.

Counseling

Psychotherapy can be delivered, to individuals, groups, or families by mental health professionals. A 2015 review found that cognitive behavioral therapy appears to be similar to antidepressant medication in terms of effect. A 2012 review found psychotherapy to be better than no treatment but not other treatments. With more complex and chronic forms of depression, a combination of medication and psychotherapy may be used. A 2014 Cochrane review found that work-directed interventions combined with clinical interventions helped to reduce sick days taken by people with depression.

Psychotherapy has been shown to be effective in older people. Successful psychotherapy appears to reduce the recurrence of depression even after it has been terminated or replaced by occasional booster sessions.

Cognitive Behavioral Therapy

Cognitive behavioral therapy (CBT) currently has the most research evidence for the treatment of depression in children and adolescents, and CBT and interpersonal psy-chotherapy (IPT) are preferred therapies for adolescent depression. In people under 18, according to the National Institute for Health and Clinical Excellence, medication should be offered only in conjunction with a psychological therapy, such as CBT, inter-personal therapy, or family therapy. Cognitive behavioral therapy has also been shown to reduce the number of sick days taken by people with depression, when used in con-junction with primary care.

The most-studied form of psychotherapy for depression is CBT, which teaches clients to challenge self-defeating, but enduring ways of thinking (cognitions) and change counter-productive behaviors. Research beginning in the mid-1990s suggested that CBT could perform as well as or better than antidepressants in patients with moder-ate to severe depression. CBT may be effective in depressed adolescents, although its effects on severe episodes are not definitively known. Several variables predict success for cognitive behavioral therapy in adolescents: higher levels of rational thoughts, less hopelessness, fewer negative thoughts, and fewer cognitive distortions. CBT is particu-larly beneficial in preventing relapse.

Cognitive behavioral therapy and occupational programs (including modification of work activities and assistance) have been shown to be effective in reducing sick days taken by workers with depression.

Variants

Several variants of cognitive behavior therapy have been used in those with de-pression, the most notable being rational emotive behavior therapy, and mindful-ness-based cognitive therapy. Mindfulness based stress reduction programs may reduce depression symptoms. Mindfulness programs also appear to be a promising intervention in youth.

Psychoanalysis

Psychoanalysis is a school of thought, founded by Sigmund Freud, which emphasizes the resolution of unconscious mental conflicts. Psychoanalytic techniques are used by some practitioners to treat clients presenting with major depression. A more widely practiced therapy, called psychodynamic psychotherapy, is in the tradition of psychoanalysis but less intensive, meeting once or twice a week. It also tends to focus more on the person's imme-diate problems, and has an additional social and interpersonal focus. In a meta-analysis of three controlled trials of Short Psychodynamic Supportive Psychotherapy, this modifica-tion was found to be as effective as medication for mild to moderate depression.

Antidepressants

Conflicting results have arisen from studies that look at the effectiveness of antidepressants in people with acute, mild to moderate depression. Stronger evidence supports the usefulness of antidepressants in the treatment of depression that is chronic (dysthymia) or severe.

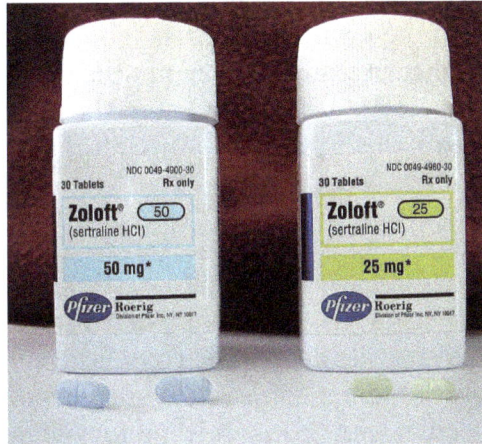

Sertraline (Zoloft) is used primarily to treat major depression in adults.

While small benefits were found, researchers Irving Kirsch and Thomas Moore state they may be due to issues with the trials rather than a true effect of the medication. In a later publication, Kirsch concluded that the overall effect of new-generation antidepressant medication is below recommended criteria for clinical significance. Similar results were obtained in a meta analysis by Fornier.

A review commissioned by the National Institute for Health and Care Excellence concluded that there is strong evidence that SSRIs have greater efficacy than placebo on achieving a 50% reduction in depression scores in moderate and severe major depression, and that there is some evidence for a similar effect in mild depression. Similarly, a Cochrane systematic review of clinical trials of the generic tricyclic antidepressant amitriptyline concluded that there is strong evidence that its efficacy is superior to placebo.

In 2014 the U.S. FDA published a systematic review of all antidepressant maintenance trials submitted to the agency between 1985 and 2012. The authors concluded that maintenance treatment reduced the risk of relapse by 52% compared to placebo, and that this effect was primarily due to recurrent depression in the placebo group rather than a drug withdrawal effect.

To find the most effective antidepressant medication with minimal side-effects, the dosages can be adjusted, and if necessary, combinations of different classes of antidepressants can be tried. Response rates to the first antidepressant administered range from 50–75%, and it can take at least six to eight weeks from the start of medication to remission. Antidepressant medication treatment is usually continued for 16 to 20 weeks after remission, to minimize the chance of recurrence, and even up to one year of continuation is recommended. People with chronic depression may need to take medication indefinitely to avoid relapse.

Selective serotonin reuptake inhibitors (SSRIs) are the primary medications prescribed, owing to their relatively mild side-effects, and because they are less toxic in overdose than other antidepressants. People who do not respond to one SSRI can be switched to another antidepressant, and this results in improvement in almost 50% of cases. Another option is to switch to the atypical antidepressant bupropion. Venlafaxine, an antidepressant with a different mechanism of action, may be modestly more effective than SSRIs. However, venlafaxine is not recommended in the UK as a first-line treatment because of evidence suggesting its risks may outweigh benefits, and it is specifically discouraged in children and adolescents.

For child and adolescent depression, fluoxetine is recommended if medication are used. Fluoxetine; however, appears to have only slight benefit in children, while other antidepressants have not been shown to be effective. There is also insufficient evidence to determine effectiveness in those with depression complicated by dementia. Any antidepressant can cause low serum sodium levels (also called hyponatremia); nevertheless, it has been reported more often with SSRIs. It is not uncommon for SSRIs to cause or worsen insomnia; the sedating antidepressant mirtazapine can be used in such cases.

Irreversible monoamine oxidase inhibitors, an older class of antidepressants, have been plagued by potentially life-threatening dietary and drug interactions. They are still used only rarely, although newer and better-tolerated agents of this class have been developed. The safety profile is different with reversible monoamine oxidase inhibitors such as moclobemide where the risk of serious dietary interactions is negligible and dietary restrictions are less strict.

For children, adolescents, and probably young adults between 18 and 24 years old, there is a higher risk of both suicidal ideations and suicidal behavior in those treated with SSRIs. For adults, it is unclear whether SSRIs affect the risk of suicidality. One review found no connection; another an increased risk; and a third no risk in those 25–65 years old and a decrease risk in those more than 65. A black box warning was introduced in the United States in 2007 on SSRI and other antidepressant medications due to increased risk of suicide in patients younger than 24 years old. Similar precautionary notice revisions were implemented by the Japanese Ministry of Health.

Other Medications

There is some evidence that omega-3 fatty acids fish oil supplements containing high levels of eicosapentaenoic acid (EPA) to docosahexaenoic acid (DHA) are effective in the treatment of, but not the prevention of major depression. However, a Cochrane review determined there was insufficient high quality evidence to suggest Omega-3 fatty acids were effective in depression. There is limited evidence that vitamin D supplementation is of value in alleviating the symptoms of depression in individuals who are vitamin D deficient. There is some preliminary evidence that COX-2 inhibitors have a beneficial effect on major depression. Lithium appears effective at lowering the risk of suicide in those with bipolar disorder and unipolar depression to nearly the same levels as the general population. There is a narrow range of effective and safe dosages of lithium thus close monitoring may be needed. Low-dose thyroid hormone may be added to existing antidepressants to treat persistent depression symptoms in people who have tried multiple courses of medication. Limited evidence suggests stimulants such as amphetamine and modafinil may be effective in the short term, or as add on therapy.

Electroconvulsive Therapy

Electroconvulsive therapy (ECT) is a standard psychiatric treatment in which seizures are electrically induced in patients to provide relief from psychiatric illnesses. ECT is used with informed consent as a last line of intervention for major depressive disorder.

A round of ECT is effective for about 50% of people with treatment-resistant major depressive disorder, whether it is unipolar or bipolar. Follow-up treatment is still poorly studied, but about half of people who respond relapse within twelve months.

Aside from effects in the brain, the general physical risks of ECT are similar to those of brief general anesthesia. Immediately following treatment, the most common adverse effects are confusion and memory loss. ECT is considered one of the least harmful treatment options available for severely depressed pregnant women.

A usual course of ECT involves multiple administrations, typically given two or three times per week until the patient is no longer suffering symptoms. ECT is administered under anesthetic with a muscle relaxant. Electroconvulsive therapy can differ in its application in three ways: electrode placement, frequency of treatments, and the electrical waveform of the stimulus. These three forms of application have significant differences in both adverse side effects and symptom remission. After treatment, drug therapy is usually continued, and some patients receive maintenance ECT.

ECT appears to work in the short term via an anticonvulsant effect mostly in the frontal lobes, and longer term via neurotrophic effects primarily in the medial temporal lobe.

Transcranial Magnetic Stimulation

Transcranial magnetic stimulation (TMS) or deep transcranial magnetic stimulation is a noninvasive method used to stimulate small regions of the brain. TMS was approved by the FDA for treatment-resistant major depressive disorder in 2008 and as of 2014 evidence supports that it is probably effective. The American Psychiatric Association the Canadian Network for Mood and Anxiety Disorders, and the Royal Australia and New Zealand College of Psychiatrists have endorsed rTMS for trMDD.

Other

Bright light therapy reduces depression symptom severity, with benefit was found for both seasonal affective disorder and for nonseasonal depression, and an effect similar to those for conventional antidepressants. For non-seasonal depression, adding light therapy to the standard antidepressant treatment was not effective. For non-seasonal depression where light was used mostly in combination with antidepressants or wake therapy a moderate effect was found, with response better than control treatment in high-quality studies, in studies that applied morning light treatment, and with people who respond to total or partial sleep deprivation. Both analyses noted poor quality, short duration, and small size of most of the reviewed studies. There is insufficient evidence for Reiki and dance movement therapy in depression.

Prognosis

Major depressive episodes often resolve over time whether or not they are treated. Outpatients on a waiting list show a 10–15% reduction in symptoms within a few months, with approximately 20% no longer meeting the full criteria for a depressive disorder. The median duration of an episode has been estimated to be 23 weeks, with the highest rate of recovery in the first three months.

Studies have shown that 80% of those suffering from their first major depressive episode will suffer from at least 1 more during their life, with a lifetime average of 4 episodes. Other general population studies indicate that around half those who have an episode recover (whether treated or not) and remain well, while the other half will have at least one more, and around 15% of those experience chronic recurrence. Studies recruiting from selective inpatient sources suggest lower recovery and higher chronicity, while studies of mostly outpatients show that nearly all recover, with a median episode duration of 11 months. Around 90% of those with severe or psychotic depression, most of whom also meet criteria for other mental disorders, experience recurrence.

Recurrence is more likely if symptoms have not fully resolved with treatment. Current guidelines recommend continuing antidepressants for four to six months after remission to prevent relapse. Evidence from many randomized controlled trials indicates continuing antidepressant medications after recovery can reduce the chance of relapse by 70% (41% on placebo vs. 18% on antidepressant). The preventive effect probably lasts for at least the first 36 months of use.

Those people experiencing repeated episodes of depression require ongoing treatment in order to prevent more severe, long-term depression. In some cases, people must take medications for long periods of time or for the rest of their lives.

Cases when outcome is poor are associated with inappropriate treatment, severe initial symptoms that may include psychosis, early age of onset, more previous episodes, incomplete recovery after 1 year, pre-existing severe mental or medical disorder, and family dysfunction as well.

Depressed individuals have a shorter life expectancy than those without depression, in part because depressed patients are at risk of dying by suicide. However, they also have a higher rate of dying from other causes, being more susceptible to medical conditions such as heart disease. Up to 60% of people who die by suicide have a mood disorder such as major depression, and the risk is especially high if a person has a marked sense of hopelessness or has both depression and borderline personality disorder. The lifetime risk of suicide associated with a diagnosis of major depression in the US is estimated at 3.4%, which averages two highly disparate figures of almost 7% for men and 1% for women (although suicide attempts are more frequent in women). The estimate is substantially lower than a previously accepted figure of 15%, which had been derived from older studies of hospitalized patients.

Depression is often associated with unemployment and poverty. Major depression is currently the leading cause of disease burden in North America and other high-income countries, and the fourth-leading cause worldwide. In the year 2030, it is predicted to be the second-leading cause of disease burden worldwide after HIV, according to the World Health Organization. Delay or failure in seeking treatment after relapse, and the failure of health professionals to provide treatment, are two barriers to reducing disability.

Epidemiology

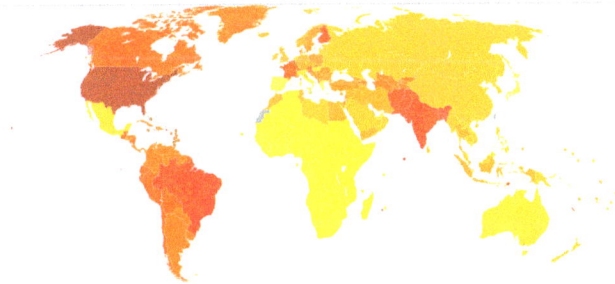

Disability-adjusted life year for unipolar depressive disorders per 100,000 inhabitants in 2004.

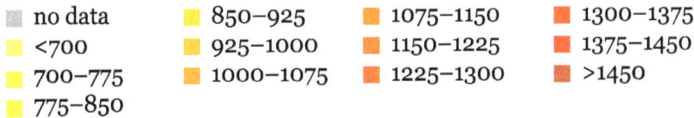

no data	850–925	1075–1150	1300–1375
<700	925–1000	1150–1225	1375–1450
700–775	1000–1075	1225–1300	>1450
775–850			

Major depressive disorder affects approximately 216 million people in 2015 (3% of the global population). The percentage of people who are affected at one point in their life varies from 7% in Japan to 21% in France. In most countries the number of people who have depression during their lives falls within an 8–18% range. In North America, the probability of having a major depressive episode within a year-long period is 3–5% for males and 8–10% for females. Major depression to be about twice as common in women as in men, although it is unclear why this is so, and whether factors unaccounted for are contributing to this. The relative increase in occurrence is related to pubertal development rather than chronological age, reaches adult ratios between the ages of 15 and 18, and appears associated with psychosocial more than hormonal factors. Depression is a major cause of disability worldwide.

People are most likely to develop their first depressive episode between the ages of 30 and 40, and there is a second, smaller peak of incidence between ages 50 and 60. The risk of major depression is increased with neurological conditions such as stroke, Parkinson's disease, or multiple sclerosis, and during the first year after childbirth. It is also more common after cardiovascular illnesses, and is related more to a poor outcome than to a better one. Studies conflict on the prevalence of depression in the elderly, but most data suggest there is a reduction in this age group. Depressive disorders are more common to observe in urban than in rural population and the prevalence is in groups with stronger socioeconomic factors i.e. homelessness.

History

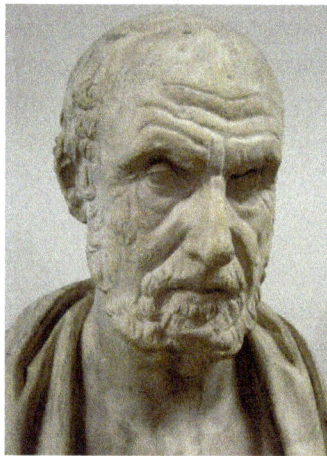

Diagnoses of depression go back at least as far as Hippocrates

The Ancient Greek physician Hippocrates described a syndrome of melancholia as a distinct disease with particular mental and physical symptoms; he characterized all "fears and despondencies, if they last a long time" as being symptomatic of the ailment. It was a similar but far broader concept than today's depression; prominence was given to a clustering of the symptoms of sadness, dejection, and despondency, and often fear, anger, delusions and obsessions were included.

The term *depression* itself was derived from the Latin verb *deprimere*, "to press down". From the 14th century, "to depress" meant to subjugate or to bring down in spirits. It was used in 1665 in English author Richard Baker's *Chronicle* to refer to someone having "a great depression of spirit", and by English author Samuel Johnson in a similar sense in 1753. The term also came into use in physiology and economics. An early usage referring to a psychiatric symptom was by French psychiatrist Louis Delasiauve in 1856, and by the 1860s it was appearing in medical dictionaries to refer to a physiological and metaphorical lowering of emotional function. Since Aristotle, melancholia had been associated with men of learning and intellectual brilliance, a hazard of contemplation and creativity. The newer concept abandoned these associations and through the 19th century, became more associated with women.

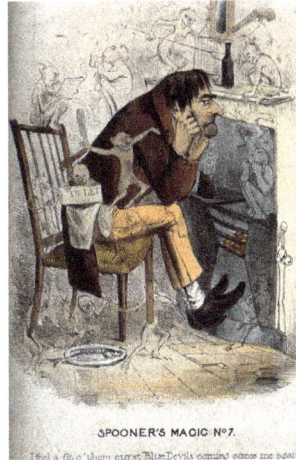

SPOONER'S MAGIC Nº 7.

A historical caricature of a man with an approaching depression

Although *melancholia* remained the dominant diagnostic term, *depression* gained increasing currency in medical treatises and was a synonym by the end of the century; German psychiatrist Emil Kraepelin may have been the first to use it as the overarching term, referring to different kinds of melancholia as *depressive states*.

Sigmund Freud likened the state of melancholia to mourning in his 1917 paper *Mourning and Melancholia*. He theorized that objective loss, such as the loss of a valued relationship through death or a romantic break-up, results in subjective loss as well; the depressed individual has identified with the object of affection through an unconscious, narcissistic process called the *libidinal cathexis* of the ego. Such loss results in severe melancholic symptoms more profound than mourning; not only is the outside world viewed negatively but the ego itself is compromised. The patient's decline of self-perception is revealed in his belief of his own blame, inferiority, and unworthiness. He also emphasized early life experiences as a predisposing factor. Adolf Meyer put forward a mixed social and biological framework emphasizing *reactions* in the context of an individual's life, and argued that the term *depression* should be used instead of *melancholia*. The first version of the DSM (DSM-I, 1952) contained *depressive reaction* and the DSM-II (1968) *depressive neurosis*, defined as an excessive reaction to internal conflict or an identifiable event, and also included a depressive type of manic-depressive psychosis within Major affective disorders.

In the mid-20th century, researchers theorized that depression was caused by a chemical imbalance in neurotransmitters in the brain, a theory based on observations made in the 1950s of the effects of reserpine and isoniazid in altering monoamine neurotransmitter levels and affecting depressive symptoms. The chemical imbalance theory has never been proven.

The term "unipolar" (along with the related term "bipolar") was coined by the neurologist and psychiatrist Karl Kleist, and subsequently used by his disciples Edda Neele and Karl Leonhard.

The term *Major depressive disorder* was introduced by a group of US clinicians in the mid-1970s as part of proposals for diagnostic criteria based on patterns of symptoms (called the "Research Diagnostic Criteria", building on earlier Feighner Criteria), and was incorporated into the DSM-III in 1980. To maintain consistency the ICD-10 used the same criteria, with only minor alterations, but using the DSM diagnostic threshold to mark a *mild depressive episode*, adding higher threshold categories for moderate and severe episodes. The ancient idea of *melancholia* still survives in the notion of a melancholic subtype.

The new definitions of depression were widely accepted, albeit with some conflicting findings and views. There have been some continued empirically based arguments for a return to the diagnosis of melancholia. There has been some criticism of the expansion of coverage of the diagnosis, related to the development and promotion of antidepressants and the biological model since the late 1950s.

Society and Culture

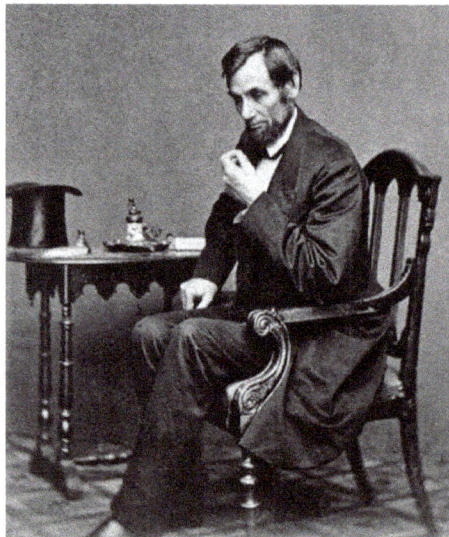

The 16th American president Abraham Lincoln had "melancholy", a condition that now may be referred to as clinical depression.

Terminology

The term "depression" is used in a number of different ways. It is often used to mean this syndrome but may refer to other mood disorders or simply to a low mood. People's conceptualizations of depression vary widely, both within and among cultures. "Because of the lack of scientific certainty," one commentator has observed, "the debate over depression turns on questions of language. What we call it—'disease,' 'disorder,' 'state of mind'—affects how we view, diagnose, and treat it." There are cultural differences in the extent to which serious depression is considered an illness requiring personal professional treatment, or is an indicator of something else, such as the need to address social or moral problems, the result of biological imbalances, or a reflection of individual differences in the understanding of distress that may reinforce feelings of powerlessness, and emotional struggle.

The diagnosis is less common in some countries, such as China. It has been argued that the Chinese traditionally deny or somatize emotional depression (although since the early 1980s, the Chinese denial of depression may have modified). Alternatively, it may be that Western cultures reframe and elevate some expressions of human distress to disorder status. Australian professor Gordon Parker and others have argued that the Western concept of depression "medicalizes" sadness or misery. Similarly, Hungarian-American psychiatrist Thomas Szasz and others argue that depression is a metaphorical illness that is inappropriately regarded as an actual disease. There has also been concern that the DSM, as well as the field of descriptive psychiatry that employs it, tends to reify abstract phenomena such as depression, which may in fact be social constructs. American archetypal psychologist James Hillman writes that depression can be healthy for the soul, insofar as "it brings refuge, limitation, focus, gravity, weight, and humble powerlessness." Hillman argues that therapeutic attempts to eliminate depression echo the Christian theme of resurrection, but have the unfortunate effect of demonizing a soulful state of being.

Stigma

Historical figures were often reluctant to discuss or seek treatment for depression due to social stigma about the condition, or due to ignorance of diagnosis or treatments. Nevertheless, analysis or interpretation of letters, journals, artwork, writings, or statements of family and friends of some historical personalities has led to the presumption that they may have had some form of depression. People who may have had depression include English author Mary Shelley, American-British writer Henry James, and American president Abraham Lincoln. Some well-known contemporary people with possible depression include Canadian songwriter Leonard Cohen and American playwright and novelist Tennessee Williams. Some pioneering psychologists, such as Americans William James and John B. Watson, dealt with their own depression.

There has been a continuing discussion of whether neurological disorders and mood disorders may be linked to creativity, a discussion that goes back to Aristotelian times. British literature gives many examples of reflections on depression. English philosopher John Stuart Mill experienced a several-months-long period of what he called "a dull state of nerves", when one is "unsusceptible to enjoyment or pleasurable excitement; one of those moods when what is pleasure at other times, becomes insipid or indifferent". He quoted English poet Samuel Taylor Coleridge's "Dejection" as a perfect description of his case: "A grief without a pang, void, dark and drear, / A drowsy, stifled, unimpassioned grief, / Which finds no natural outlet or relief / In word, or sigh, or tear." English writer Samuel Johnson used the term "the black dog" in the 1780s to describe his own depression, and it was subsequently popularized by depression sufferer former British Prime Minister Sir Winston Churchill.

Social stigma of major depression is widespread, and contact with mental health services reduces this only slightly. Public opinions on treatment differ markedly to those of health professionals; alternative treatments are held to be more helpful than pharmacological ones, which are viewed poorly. In the UK, the Royal College of Psychiatrists and the Royal College of General Practitioners conducted a joint Five-year Defeat Depression campaign to educate and reduce stigma from 1992 to 1996; a MORI study conducted afterwards showed a small positive change in public attitudes to depression and treatment.

Research

Trials are looking at the effects of botulinum toxins on depression. The idea is that the drug is used to make the person look less frowning and that this stops the negative facial feedback from the face. In 2015 it turned out, however, that the partly positive effects that had been observed until then could have been placebo effects.

MDD has been studied by taking MRI scans of patients with depression have revealed a number of differences in brain structure compared to those who are not depressed. Meta-analyses of neuroimaging studies in major depression reported that, compared to controls, depressed patients had increased volume of the lateral ventricles and adrenal gland and smaller volumes of the basal ganglia, thalamus, hippocampus, and frontal lobe (including the orbitofrontal cortex and gyrus rectus). Hyperintensities have been associated with patients with a late age of onset, and have led to the development of the theory of vascular depression.

Elderly

Depression is especially common among those over 65 years of age and increases in frequency with age beyond this age. In addition the risk of depression increases in relation to the age and frailty of the individual. Depression is one the most important factors which negatively impact quality of life in adults as well as the elderly. Both symptoms and treatment among the elderly differ from those of the rest of the adult populations.

As with many other diseases it is common among the elderly not to present classical depressive symptoms. Diagnosis and treatment is further complicated in that the elderly are often simultaneously treated with a number of other drugs, and often have other concurrent diseases. Treatment differs in that studies of SSRI-drugs have shown lesser and often inadequate effect among the elderly, while other drugs with more clear effects have adverse effects which can be especially difficult to handle among the elderly. Duloxetine is an SNRI-drug with documented effect on recurring depression among the elderly, but has adverse effects in form of dizziness, dryness of the mouth, diarrhea, and constipation.

Problem solving therapy was as of 2015 the only psychological therapy with proven effect, and can be likened to a simpler form of cognitive behavioral therapy. However, elderly with depression are seldom offered any psychological treatment, and the evidence surrounding which other treatments are effective is incomplete. Electroconvulsive therapy (ECT or electric-shock therapy) has been used as treatment of the elderly, and register-studies suggest it is effective although less so among the elderly than among the rest of the adult population.

The risks involved with treatment of depression among the elderly as opposed to benefits is not entirely clear. Awaiting more evidence on how depression-treatment among the elderly is best designed it is important to follow up treatment results, and to reconsider changing treatments if it does not help.

Other Animals

Models of depression in animals for the purpose of study include iatrogenic depression models (such as drug induced), forced swim tests, tail suspension test, and learned helplessness models. Criteria frequently used to assess depression in animals include expression of despair, neurovegetative changes, and anhedonia, as many other depressive criteria are untestable in animals such as guilt and suicidality.

Bipolar Disorder

Bipolar disorder, previously known as manic depression, is a mental disorder that causes periods of depression and periods of elevated mood. The elevated mood is significant and is known as mania or hypomania, depending on its severity, or whether symptoms of psychosis are present. During mania, an individual behaves or feels abnormally energetic, happy, or irritable. Individuals often make poorly thought out decisions with little regard to the consequences. The need for sleep is usually reduced during manic phases. During periods of depression, there may be crying, a negative outlook on life, and poor eye contact with others. The risk of suicide among those with the illness is high at greater than 6 percent over 20 years, while self-harm occurs in 30–40 percent. Other mental health issues such as anxiety disorders and substance use disorder are commonly associated.

The causes are not clearly understood, but both environmental and genetic factors play a role. Many genes of small effect contribute to risk. Environmental factors include a history of childhood abuse, and long-term stress. The condition is divided into bipolar

I disorder if there has been at least one manic episode, with or without depressive episodes, and bipolar II disorder if there has been at least one hypomanic episode (but no manic episodes) and one major depressive episode. In those with less severe symptoms of a prolonged duration, the condition cyclothymic disorder may be diagnosed. If due to drugs or medical problems, it is classified separately. Other conditions that may present in a similar manner include attention deficit hyperactivity disorder, personality disorders, schizophrenia, and substance use disorder as well as a number of medical conditions. Medical testing is not required for a diagnosis, though blood tests or medical imaging can be done to rule out other problems.

Treatment commonly includes psychotherapy, as well as medications such as mood stabilizers and antipsychotics. Examples of mood stabilizers that are commonly used include lithium and various anticonvulsants. Treatment in a hospital without the individual's consent may be required if a person is at risk to themselves or others but refuses treatment. Severe behavioral problems may be managed with short term antipsychotics or benzodiazepines. In periods of mania it is recommended that antidepressants be stopped. If antidepressants are used for periods of depression they should be used with a mood stabilizer. Electroconvulsive therapy (ECT), while not very well studied, may be helpful for those who do not respond to other treatments. If treatments are stopped, it is recommended that this be done slowly. Many individuals have financial, social or work-related problems due to the illness. These difficulties occur a quarter to a third of the time on average. The risk of death from natural causes such as heart disease is twice that of the general population. This is due to poor lifestyle choices and the side effects from medications.

Bipolar disorder affects approximately 1% of the global population. The most common age at which symptoms begin is 25. Rates appear to be similar in females and males. The economic costs of the disorder has been estimated at $45 billion for the United States in 1991. A large proportion of this was related to a higher number of missed work days, estimated at 50 per year. People with bipolar disorder often face problems with social stigma.

Signs and Symptoms

Mania is the defining feature of bipolar disorder and can occur with different levels of severity. With milder levels of mania, known as hypomania, individuals are energetic, excitable, and may be highly productive. As hypomania worsens, individuals begin to exhibit erratic and impulsive behavior, often making poor decisions due to unrealistic ideas about the future, and sleep very reduced. At the extreme, manic individuals can experience distorted or delusional beliefs about the universe, hallucinate, hear voices, to the point of psychosis. A depressive episode commonly follows an episode of mania. The biological mechanisms responsible for switching from a manic or hypomanic episode to a depressive episode, or vice versa, remain poorly understood.

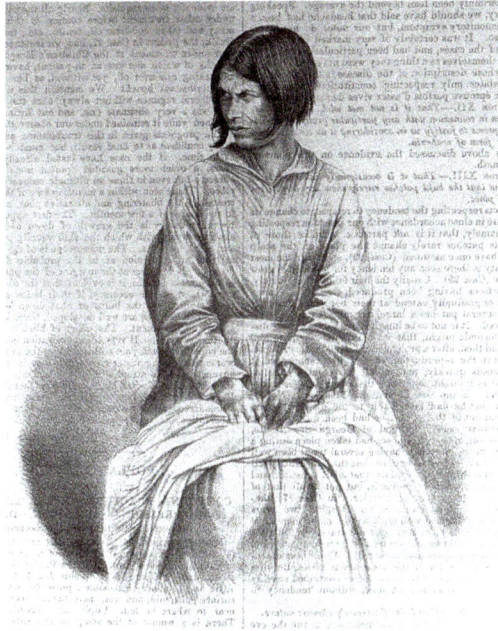
An 1858 lithograph captioned 'Melancholy passing into mania'.

Manic Episodes

Mania is a distinct period of at least one week of elevated or irritable mood, which can range from euphoria to delirium, and those experiencing hypo- or mania may exhibit three or more of the following behaviors: speak in a rapid, uninterruptible manner, short attention span, racing thoughts, increased goal-oriented activities, agitation, or they may exhibit behaviors characterized as impulsive or high-risk, such as hypersexuality or excessive spending. To meet the definition for a manic episode, these behaviors must impair the individual's ability to socialize or work. If untreated, a manic episode usually lasts three to six months.

People with hypomania or mania may experience a decreased need of sleep, speak excessively in addition to speaking rapidly, and impaired judgment. Manic individuals often have a history of substance abuse developed over years as a form of "self-medication". At the more extreme, a person in a full blown manic state can experience psychosis; a break with reality, a state in which thinking is affected along with mood. They may feel unstoppable, or as if they have been "chosen" and are on a "special mission", or have other grandiose or delusional ideas. This may lead to violent behavior and, sometimes, hospitalization in an inpatient psychiatric hospital. The severity of manic symptoms can be measured by rating scales such as the Young Mania Rating Scale, though questions remain about their reliability.

The onset of a manic (or depressive) episode is often foreshadowed by sleep disturbances. Mood changes, psychomotor and appetite changes, and an increase in anxiety can also occur up to three weeks before a manic episode develops.

Hypomanic Episodes

Hypomania is the milder form of mania, defined as at least four days of the same criteria as mania, but does not cause a significant decrease in the individual's ability to socialize or work, lacks psychotic features such as delusions or hallucinations, and does not require psychiatric hospitalization. Overall functioning may actually increase during episodes of hypomania and is thought to serve as a defense mechanism against depression by some. Hypomanic episodes rarely progress to full blown manic episodes. Some people who experience hypomania show increased creativity while others are irritable or demonstrate poor judgment.

Hypomania may feel good to some persons who experience it, though most people who experience hypomania state that the stress of the experience is very painful. Bipolar people who go hypo, however, tend to forget the effects of their actions on those around them. Even when family and friends recognize mood swings, the individual will often deny that anything is wrong. What might be called a "hypomanic event", if not accompanied by depressive episodes, is often not deemed problematic, unless the mood changes are uncontrollable, volatile or mercurial. Most commonly, symptoms continue for a few weeks to a few months.

Depressive Episodes

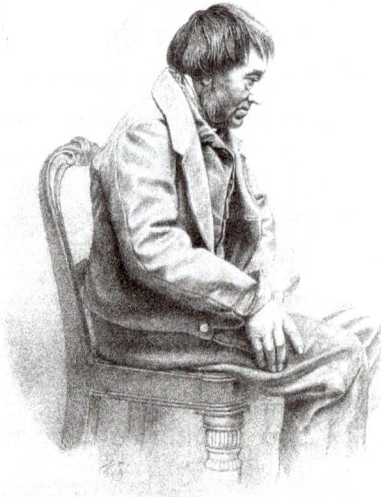

'Melancholy' by W. Bagg after a photograph by Hugh Welch Diamond

Symptoms of the depressive phase of bipolar disorder include persistent feelings of sadness, irritability or anger, loss of interest in previously enjoyed activities, excessive or inappropriate guilt, hopelessness, sleeping too much or not enough, changes in appetite and/or weight, fatigue, problems concentrating, self-loathing or feelings of worthlessness, and thoughts of death or suicidal ideation. In severe cases, the individual may develop symptoms of psychosis, a condition also known as severe bipolar disorder with psychotic features. These symptoms include delusions and hallucinations. A major depressive episode persists for at least two weeks, and may result in suicide if left untreated.

The earlier the age of onset, the more likely the first few episodes are to be depressive. Because a bipolar diagnosis requires a manic or hypomanic episode, many patients are initially diagnosed and treated as having major depression and then incorrectly prescribed antidepressants.

Mixed Affective Episodes

In bipolar disorder, mixed state is a condition during which symptoms of both mania and depression occur simultaneously. Individuals experiencing a mixed state may have manic symptoms such as grandiose thoughts while simultaneously experiencing depressive symptoms such as excessive guilt or feeling suicidal. Mixed states are considered to be high-risk for suicidal behavior since depressive emotions such as hopelessness are often paired with mood swings or difficulties with impulse control. Anxiety disorder occurs more frequently as a comorbidity in mixed bipolar episodes than in non-mixed bipolar depression or mania. Substance abuse (including alcohol) also follows this trend, thereby appearing to depict bipolar symptoms as no more than a consequence of substance abuse.

Associated Features

Associated features are clinical phenomena that often accompany the disorder but are not part of the diagnostic criteria. In adults with the condition, bipolar disorder is often accompanied by changes in cognitive processes and abilities. These include reduced attentional and executive capabilities and impaired memory. How the individual processes the universe also depends on the phase of the disorder, with differential characteristics between the manic, hypomanic and depressive states. Some studies have found a significant association between bipolar disorder and creativity. Those with bipolar disorder may have difficulty in maintaining relationships. There are several common childhood precursors seen in children who later receive a diagnosis of bipolar disorder; these disorders include mood abnormalities, full major depressive episodes, and attention deficit hyperactivity disorder (ADHD).

Comorbid Conditions

The diagnosis of bipolar disorder can be complicated by coexisting (comorbid) psychiatric conditions including the following: obsessive-compulsive disorder, substance abuse, eating disorders, attention deficit hyperactivity disorder, social phobia, premenstrual syndrome (including premenstrual dysphoric disorder), or panic disorder. A careful longitudinal analysis of symptoms and episodes, enriched if possible by discussions with friends and family members, is crucial to establishing a treatment plan where these comorbidities exist.

Causes

The causes of bipolar disorder likely vary between individuals and the exact mechanism underlying the disorder remains unclear. Genetic influences are believed to account for 60–80 percent of the risk of developing the disorder indicating a strong hereditary component. The overall heritability of the bipolar spectrum has been estimated at 0.71. Twin studies have been limited by relatively small sample sizes but have indicated a substantial genetic contribution, as well as environmental influence. For bipolar disorder type I, the (probandwise) concordance rates in modern studies have been consistently estimated at around 40 percent in identical twins (same genes), compared to about 5 percent in fraternal twins. A combination of bipolar I, II and cyclothymia produced concordance rates of 42 percent vs. 11 percent, with a relatively lower ratio for bipolar II that likely reflects heterogeneity. There is overlap with unipolar depression and if this is also counted in the co-twin the concordance with bipolar disorder rises to 67 percent in monozygotic twins and 19 percent in dizygotic. The relatively low concordance between dizygotic twins brought up together suggests that shared family environmental effects are limited, although the ability to detect them has been limited by small sample sizes.

Genetic

Behavioral genetic studies have suggested that many chromosomal regions and candidate genes are related to bipolar disorder susceptibility with each gene exerting a mild to moderate effect. The risk of bipolar disorder is nearly ten-fold higher in first degree-relatives of those affected with bipolar disorder when compared to the general population; similarly, the risk of major depressive disorder is three times higher in relatives of those with bipolar disorder when compared to the general population.

Although the first genetic linkage finding for mania was in 1969, the linkage studies have been inconsistent. The largest and most recent genome-wide association study failed to find any particular locus that exerts a large effect reinforcing the idea that no single gene is responsible for bipolar disorder in most cases.

Findings point strongly to heterogeneity, with different genes being implicated in different families. Robust and replicable genome-wide significant associations showed several common single nucleotide polymorphisms, including variants within the genes CACNA1C, ODZ4, and NCAN.

Advanced paternal age has been linked to a somewhat increased chance of bipolar disorder in offspring, consistent with a hypothesis of increased new genetic mutations.

Physiological

Abnormalities in the structure and/or function of certain brain circuits could underlie bipolar. Meta-analyses of structural MRI studies in bipolar disorder report an increase in the volume of the lateral ventricles, globus pallidus and increase in the rates of deep white matter hyperintensities. Functional MRI findings suggest that abnormal modulation between ventral prefrontal and limbic regions, especially the amygdala, are likely contribute to poor emotional regulation and mood symptoms.

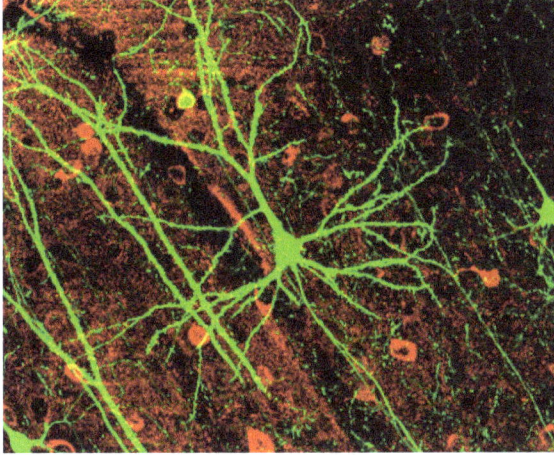

Brain imaging studies have revealed differences in the volume of various brain regions between BD patients and healthy control subjects

Euthymic bipolar people show decreased activity in the lingual gyrus, while people who are manic demonstrated decreased activity in the inferior frontal cortex, while no differences were found in people with depressed bipolar. People with bipolar have increased activation of left hemisphere ventral limbic areas and decreased activation of right hemisphere cortical structures related to cognition.

One proposed model for bipolar suggests that hypersensitivity of reward circuits consisting of fronto-striatal circuits causes mania and hyposensitivity of these circuits cause depression.

According to the "kindling" hypothesis, when people who are genetically predisposed toward bipolar disorder experience stressful events, the stress threshold at which mood changes occur becomes progressively lower, until the episodes eventually start (and recur) spontaneously. There is evidence supporting an association between early-life stress and dysfunction of the hypothalamic-pituitary-adrenal axis (HPA axis) leading to its over activation, which may play a role in the pathogenesis of bipolar disorder.

Other brain components which have been proposed to play a role are the mitochondria and a sodium ATPase pump. Circadian rhythms and melatonin activity also seem to be altered.

Environmental

Environmental factors play a significant role in the development and course of bipolar disorder, and individual psychosocial variables may interact with genetic dispositions.

It is probable that recent life events and interpersonal relationships contribute to the onset and recurrence of bipolar mood episodes, just as they do for unipolar depression. In surveys, 30–50 percent of adults diagnosed with bipolar disorder report traumatic/abusive experiences in childhood, which is associated on average with earlier onset, a higher rate of suicide attempts, and more co-occurring disorders such as PTSD. The number of reported stressful events in childhood is higher in those with an adult diagnosis of bipolar spectrum disorder compared to those without, particularly events stemming from a harsh environment rather than from the child's own behavior.

Neurological

Less commonly bipolar disorder, or a bipolar-like disorder, may occur as a result of or in association with a neurological condition or injury. Such conditions and injuries include (but are not limited to) stroke, traumatic brain injury, HIV infection, multiple sclerosis, porphyria, and rarely temporal lobe epilepsy.

Neurochemical

Dopamine, a known neurotransmitter responsible for mood cycling, has been shown to have increased transmission during the manic phase. The dopamine hypothesis states that the increase in dopamine results in secondary homeostatic down regulation of key systems and receptors such as an increase in dopamine mediated G protein-coupled receptors. This results in decreased dopamine transmission characteristic of the depressive phase. The depressive phase ends with homeostatic up regulation potentially restarting the cycle over again.

Glutamate is significantly increased within the left dorsolateral prefrontal cortex during the manic phase of bipolar disorder, and returns to normal levels once the phase is over. The increase in GABA is possibly caused by a disturbance in early development causing a disturbance of cell migration and the formation of normal lamination, the layering of brain structures commonly associated with the cerebral cortex.

Medications use to treat bipolar may exert their effect by modulating intracellular signaling, such as through depleting myo-inositol levels, inhibition of cAMP signaling, and through altering G coupled proteins

Decreased levels of 5-HIAA in the CSF of bipolar patients during both depressed and manic phases. Increased dopaminergic activity has been hypothesized in manic states due to the ability of dopamine agonist to stimulant mania in bipolar patients. Decreased sensitivity of regulatory a2 adrenergic receptors as well as increased cell counts in the locus coeruleus indicated increased noradrenergic activity in manic patients. Low plasma GABA levels on both sides of the mood spectrum have been found. One review found no difference in monoamine levels, but found abnormal norepinephrine turnover in bipolar patients. Tyrosine depletion was found to attenuate the effects of methamphetamine in bipolar patients as well as symptoms of mania, implicating dopamine in mania. VMAT2 binding was found to be increased in one study of bipolar manic patients.

Pathophysiology

Bipolar disorder has also been linked to decreased volume in certain areas of the hippocampus, which is the part of the brain for memory processing.

Prevention

Attempts at prevention of bipolar disorder have focused on stress (such as childhood adversity or highly conflictual families) which, although not a diagnostically specific causal agent for bipolar, does place genetically and biologically vulnerable individuals at risk for a more pernicious course of illness. There has been debate regarding the causal relationship between usage of cannabis and bipolar disorder.

Diagnosis

Bipolar disorder is commonly diagnosed during adolescence or early adulthood, but onset can occur throughout the life cycle. The disorder can be difficult to distinguish from unipolar depression and the average delay in diagnosis is 5–10 years after symptoms begin. Diagnosis of bipolar disorder takes several factors into account and considers the self-reported experiences of the symptomatic individual, abnormal behavior reported by family members, friends or co-workers, observable signs of illness as assessed by a clinician, and often a medical work-up to rule-out medical causes. In diagnosis, caregiver-scored rating scales, specifically the mother, has been found to be more accurate than teacher and youth report in predicting identifying youths with bipolar disorder. Assessment is usually done on an outpatient basis; admission to an inpatient facility is considered if there is a risk to oneself or others. The most widely used criteria for diagnosing bipolar disorder are from the American Psychiatric Association's (APA) *Diagnostic and Statistical Manual of Mental Disorders*, Fifth Edition (DSM-5) and the World Health Organization's (WHO) *International Statistical Classification of Diseases and Related Health Problems*, 10th Edition (ICD-10). The ICD-10 criteria are used more often in clinical settings outside of the U.S. while the DSM criteria are used clinically within the U.S. and are the prevailing criteria used internationally in research studies. The DSM-5, published in 2013, included further and more accurate specifiers compared to its predecessor, the DSM-IV-TR. Semi structured interviews such as the Kiddie Schedule for Affective Disorders and Schizophrenia (KSADS) and the Structured Clinical Interview for DSM-IV (SCID) are used for diagnostic confirmation of bipolar disorder.

Several rating scales for the screening and evaluation of bipolar disorder exist, including the Bipolar spectrum diagnostic scale, Mood Disorder Questionnaire, the General Behavior Inventory and the Hypomania Checklist. The use of evaluation scales can not substitute a full clinical interview but they serve to systematize the recollection of symptoms. On the other hand, instruments for screening bipolar disorder tend to have lower sensitivity.

Differential diagnosis

There are several other mental disorders with symptoms similar to those seen in bipolar disorder. These disorders include schizophrenia, major depressive disorder, attention deficit hyperactivity disorder (ADHD), and certain personality disorders, such as borderline personality disorder.

Although there are no biological tests that are diagnostic of bipolar disorder, blood tests and/or imaging may be carried out to exclude medical illnesses with clinical presentations similar to that of bipolar disorder such as hypothyroidism or hyperthyroidism, metabolic disturbance, a chronic disease, or an infection such as HIV or syphilis. A review of current and recent medications and drug use is considered to rule out these causes; common medications that can cause manic symptoms include antidepressants, prednisone, Parkinson's disease medications, thyroid hormone, stimulants (including cocaine and methamphetamine), and certain antibiotics. An EEG may be used to exclude neurological disorders such as epilepsy, and a CT scan or MRI of the head may be used to exclude brain lesions. Additional testing is especially indicated when age of first onset is mid to late life. Investigations are not generally repeated for a relapse unless there is a specific medical indication.

Bipolar spectrum

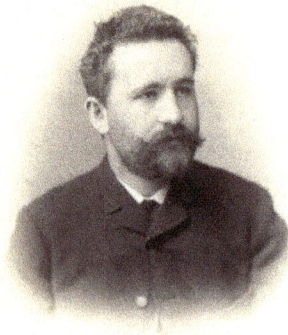

Since Emil Kraepelin's distinction between bipolar disorder and schizophrenia in the 19th century, researchers have defined a spectrum of different types of bipolar disorder

Bipolar spectrum disorders includes: bipolar I disorder, bipolar II disorder, cyclothymic disorder and cases where subthreshold symptoms are found to cause clinically significant impairment or distress. These disorders involve major depressive episodes that alternate with manic or hypomanic episodes, or with mixed episodes that feature symptoms of both mood states. The concept of the bipolar spectrum is similar to that of Emil Kraepelin's original concept of manic depressive illness.

Unipolar hypomania without accompanying depression has been noted in the medical literature. There is speculation as to whether this condition may occur with greater frequency in the general, untreated population; successful social function of these potentially high-achieving individuals may lead to being labeled as normal, rather than as individuals with substantial dysregulation.

Criteria and subtypes

The DSM and the ICD characterize bipolar disorder as a spectrum of disorders occurring on a continuum. The DSM-5 lists three specific subtypes:

- Bipolar I disorder: At least one manic episode is necessary to make the diagnosis; depressive episodes are common in the vast majority of cases with bipolar disorder I, but are unnecessary for the diagnosis. Specifiers such as "mild, moderate, moderate-severe, severe" and "with psychotic features" should be added as applicable to indicate the presentation and course of the disorder.

- Bipolar II disorder: No manic episodes and one or more hypomanic episodes and one or more major depressive episode. Hypomanic episodes do not go to the full extremes of mania (*i.e.*, do not usually cause severe social or occupational impairment, and are without psychosis), and this can make bipolar II more difficult to diagnose, since the hypomanic episodes may simply appear as periods of successful high productivity and are reported less frequently than a distressing, crippling depression.

- Cyclothymia: A history of hypomanic episodes with periods of depression that do not meet criteria for major depressive episodes.

When relevant, specifiers for *peripartum onset* and *with rapid cycling* should be used with any subtype. Individuals who have subthreshold symptoms that cause clinically significant distress or impairment, but do not meet full criteria for one of the three subtypes may be diagnosed with other specified or unspecified bipolar disorder. Other specified bipolar disorder is used when a clinician chooses to provide an explanation for why the full criteria were not met (e.g., hypomania without a prior major depressive episode).

Rapid Cycling

Most people who meet criteria for bipolar disorder experience a number of episodes, on average 0.4 to 0.7 per year, lasting three to six months. *Rapid cycling*, however, is a course specifier that may be applied to any of the above subtypes. It is defined as having four or more mood disturbance episodes within a one-year span and is found in a significant proportion of individuals with bipolar disorder. These episodes are separated from each other by a remission (partial or full) for at least two months or a switch in mood polarity (i.e., from a depressive episode to a manic episode or vice versa). The definition of rapid cycling most frequently cited in the literature (including the DSM) is that of Dunner and Fieve: at least four major depressive, manic, hypomanic or mixed episodes are required to have occurred during a 12-month period. Ultra-rapid (days) and ultra-ultra rapid or ultradian (within a day) cycling have also been described. The literature examining the pharmacological treatment of rapid cycling is sparse and there is no clear consensus with respect to its optimal pharmacological management.

Management

There are a number of pharmacological and psychotherapeutic techniques used to treat bipolar disorder. Individuals may use self-help and pursue recovery.

Hospitalization may be required especially with the manic episodes present in bipolar I. This can be voluntary or (if mental health legislation allows and varying state-to-state regulations in the USA) involuntary (called civil or involuntary commitment). Long-term inpatient stays are now less common due to deinstitutionalization, although these can still occur. Following (or in lieu of) a hospital admission, support services available can include drop-in centers, visits from members of a community mental health team or an Assertive Community Treatment team, supported employment and patient-led support groups, intensive outpatient programs. These are sometimes referred to as partial-inpatient programs.

Psychosocial

Psychotherapy is aimed at alleviating core symptoms, recognizing episode triggers, reducing negative expressed emotion in relationships, recognizing prodromal symptoms before full-blown recurrence, and, practicing the factors that lead to maintenance of remission. Cognitive behavioral therapy, family-focused therapy, and psychoeducation have the most evidence for efficacy in regard to relapse prevention, while interpersonal and social rhythm therapy and cognitive-behavioral therapy appear the most effective in regard to residual depressive symptoms. Most studies have been based only on bipolar I, however, and treatment during the acute phase can be a particular challenge. Some clinicians emphasize the need to talk with individuals experiencing mania, to develop a therapeutic alliance in support of recovery.

Medication

A number of medications are used to treat bipolar disorder. The medication with the best evidence is lithium, which is effective in treating acute manic episodes and preventing relapses; lithium is also an effective treatment for bipolar depression. Lithium reduces the risk of suicide, self-harm, and death in people with bipolar disorder. It is unclear if ketamine is useful in bipolar as of 2015.

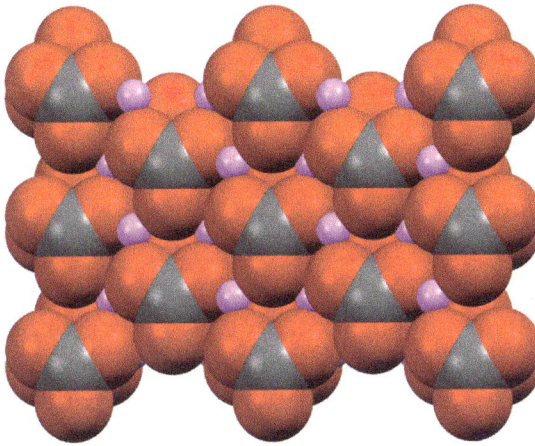

Lithium carbonate is one of many treatments for bipolar disorder

Four anticonvulsants are used in the treatment of bipolar disorder. Carbamazepine effectively treats manic episodes, with some evidence it has greater benefit in rapid-cycling bipolar disorder, or those with more psychotic symptoms or a more schizoaffective clinical picture. It is less effective in preventing relapse than lithium or valproate. Carbamazepine became a popular treatment option for bipolar in the late 1980s and early 1990s, but was displaced by sodium valproate in the 1990s. Since then, valproate has become a commonly prescribed treatment, and is effective in treating manic episodes. Lamotrigine has some efficacy in treating bipolar depression, and this benefit is greatest in more severe depression. It has also been shown to have some benefit in preventing further episodes, though there are concerns about the studies done, and is of no benefit in rapid cycling disorder. The effectiveness of topiramate is unknown. Depending on the severity of the case, anticonvulsants may be used in combination with lithium or on their own.

Antipsychotic medications are effective for short-term treatment of bipolar manic episodes and appear to be superior to lithium and anticonvulsants for this purpose. However, other medications such as lithium are preferred for long-term use. Olanzapine is effective in preventing relapses, although the evidence is not as solid as the evidence for lithium. Antidepressants have not been found to be of any benefit over that found with mood stabilizers. Furthermore, antidepressants are not recommended for use alone in the treatment of bipolar disorder.

Short courses of benzodiazepines may be used in addition to other medications until mood stabilizing become effective. Electroconvulsive therapy (ECT) is an effective form of treatment for acute mood disturbances in those with bipolar disorder, especially when psychotic or catatonic features are displayed. ECT is also recommended for use in pregnant women with bipolar disorder.

Alternative Medicine

Several studies have suggested that omega 3 fatty acids may have beneficial effects on depressive symptoms, but not manic symptoms. However, only a few small studies of variable quality have been published and there is not enough evidence to draw any firm conclusions.

Prognosis

A lifelong condition with periods of partial or full recovery in between recurrent episodes of relapse, bipolar disorder is considered to be a major health problem worldwide because of the increased rates of disability and premature mortality. It is also associated with co-occurring psychiatric and medical problems and high rates of initial under- or misdiagnosis, causing a delay in appropriate treatment interventions and contributing to poorer prognoses. After a diagnosis is made, it remains difficult to achieve complete remission of all symptoms with the currently available psychiatric medications and symptoms often become progressively more severe over time.

Compliance with medications is one of the most significant factors that can decrease the rate and severity of relapse and have a positive impact on overall prognosis. However, the types of medications used in treating BD commonly cause side effects and more than 75% of individuals with BD inconsistently take their medications for various reasons.

Of the various types of the disorder, rapid cycling (four or more episodes in one year) is associated with the worst prognosis due to higher rates of self-harm and suicide. Individuals diagnosed with bipolar who have a family history of bipolar disorder are at a greater risk for more frequent manic/hypomanic episodes. Early onset and psychotic features are also associated with worse outcomes, as well as subtypes that are nonresponsive to lithium.

Early recognition and intervention also improve prognosis as the symptoms in earlier stages are less severe and more responsive to treatment. Onset after adolescence is connected to better prognoses for both genders, and being male is a protective factor against higher levels of depression. For women, better social functioning prior to developing bipolar disorder and being a parent are protective towards suicide attempts.

Functioning

People with bipolar disorder often experience a decline in cognitive functioning during (or possibly before) their first episode, after which a certain degree of cognitive dysfunction typically becomes permanent, with more severe impairment during acute phases and moderate impairment during periods of remission. As a result, two-thirds of people with BD continue to experience impaired psychosocial functioning in between episodes even when their mood symptoms are in full remission. A similar pattern in seen in both BD-I and BD-II, but people with BD-II experience a lesser degree of impairment. Cognitive deficits typically increase over the course of the illness. Higher degrees of impairment correlate with the number of previous manic episodes and hospitalizations, and with the presence psychotic symptoms. Early intervention can slow the progression of cognitive impairment, while treatment at later stages can help reduce distress and negative consequences related to cognitive dysfunction.

Despite the overly ambitious goals that are frequently part of manic episodes, symptoms of mania undermine the ability to achieve these goals and often interfere an individual's social and occupational functioning. One third of people with BD remain unemployed for one year following a hospitalization for mania. Depressive symptoms during and between episodes, which occur much more frequently for most people than hypomanic or manic symptoms over the course of illness, are associated with lower functional recovery in between episodes, including unemployment or underemployment for both BD-I and BD-II. However, the course of illness (duration, age of onset, number of hospitalizations, and presence or not of rapid cycling) and cognitive performance are the best predictors of employment outcomes in individuals with bipolar disorder, followed by symptoms of depression and years of education.

Recovery and Recurrence

A naturalistic study from first admission for mania or mixed episode (representing the hospitalized and therefore most severe cases) found that 50 percent achieved syndromal recovery (no longer meeting criteria for the diagnosis) within six weeks and 98 percent within two years. Within two years, 72 percent achieved symptomatic recovery (no symptoms at all) and 43 percent achieved functional recovery (regaining of prior occupational and residential status). However, 40 percent went on to experience a new episode of mania or depression within 2 years of syndromal recovery, and 19 percent switched phases without recovery.

Symptoms preceding a relapse (prodromal), specially those related to mania, can be reliably identified by people with bipolar disorder. There have been intents to teach patients coping strategies when noticing such symptoms with encouraging results.

Suicide

Bipolar disorder can cause suicidal ideation that leads to suicidal attempts. Individuals whose bipolar disorder begins with a depressive or mixed affective episode seem to have a poorer prognosis and an increased risk of suicide. One out of two people with bipolar disorder attempt suicide at least once during their lifetime and many attempts are successfully completed. The annual average suicide rate is 0.4 percent, which is 10–20 times that of the general population. The standardized mortality ratio from suicide in bipolar disorder is between 18 and 25. The lifetime risk of suicide has been estimated to be as high as 20 percent in those with bipolar disorder.

Epidemiology

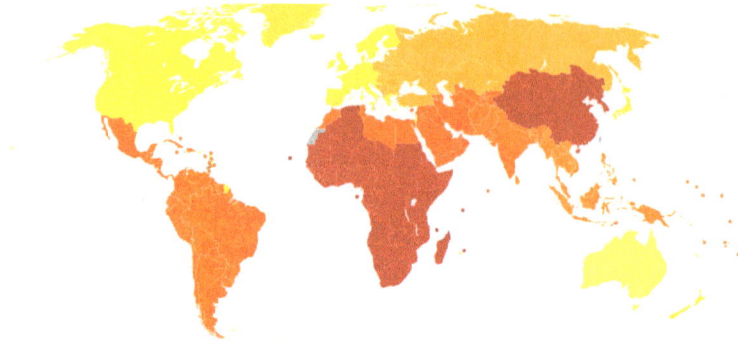

Burden of bipolar disorder around the world: disability-adjusted life years per 100,000 inhabitants in 2004.

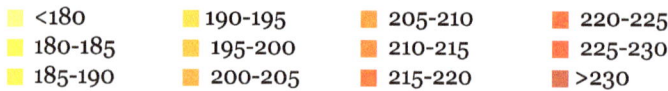

<180	190-195	205-210	220-225
180-185	195-200	210-215	225-230
185-190	200-205	215-220	>230

Bipolar disorder is the sixth leading cause of disability worldwide and has a lifetime prevalence of about 3 percent in the general population. However, a reanalysis of data from the National Epidemiological Catchment Area survey in the United States suggested that 0.8 percent of the population experience a manic episode at least once (the diagnostic threshold for bipolar I) and a further 0.5 percent have a hypomanic episode (the diagnostic threshold for bipolar II or cyclothymia). Including sub-threshold diagnostic criteria, such as one or two symptoms over a short time-period, an additional 5.1 percent of the population, adding up to a total of 6.4 percent, were classified as having a bipolar spectrum disorder. A more recent analysis of data from a second US National Comorbidity Survey found that 1 percent met lifetime prevalence criteria for bipolar I, 1.1 percent for bipolar II, and 2.4 percent for subthreshold symptoms.

There are conceptual and methodological limitations and variations in the findings. Prevalence studies of bipolar disorder are typically carried out by lay interviewers who follow fully structured/fixed interview schemes; responses to single items from such interviews may suffer limited validity. In addition, diagnoses (and therefore estimates of prevalence) vary depending on whether a categorical or spectrum approach is used. This consideration has led to concerns about the potential for both underdiagnosis and overdiagnosis.

The incidence of bipolar disorder is similar in men and women as well as across different cultures and ethnic groups. A 2000 study by the World Health Organization found that prevalence and incidence of bipolar disorder are very similar across the world. Age-standardized prevalence per 100,000 ranged from 421.0 in South Asia to 481.7 in Africa and Europe for men and from 450.3 in Africa and Europe to 491.6 in Oceania for women. However, severity may differ widely across the globe. Disability-adjusted life year rates, for example, appear to be higher in developing countries, where medical coverage may be poorer and medication less available. Within the United States, Asian

Americans have significantly lower rates than their African and European American counterparts.

Late adolescence and early adulthood are peak years for the onset of bipolar disorder. One study also found that in 10 percent of bipolar cases, the onset of mania had happened after the patient had turned 50.

History

Variations in moods and energy levels have been observed as part of the human experience since throughout history. The words "melancholia", an old word for depression, and "mania" originated in Ancient Greece. The word melancholia is derived from *melas*, meaning black, and *chole*, meaning bile or gall, indicative of the term's origins in pre-Hippocratic humoral theory. Within the humoral theories, mania was viewed as arising from an excess of yellow bile, or a mixture of black and yellow bile. The linguistic origins of mania, however, are not so clear-cut. Several etymologies were proposed by the Ancient Roman physician Caelius Aurelianus, including the Greek word *ania*, meaning "to produce great mental anguish", and *manos*, meaning "relaxed" or "loose", which would contextually approximate to an excessive relaxing of the mind or soul. There are at least five other candidates, and part of the confusion surrounding the exact etymology of the word mania is its varied usage in the pre-Hippocratic poetry and mythology.

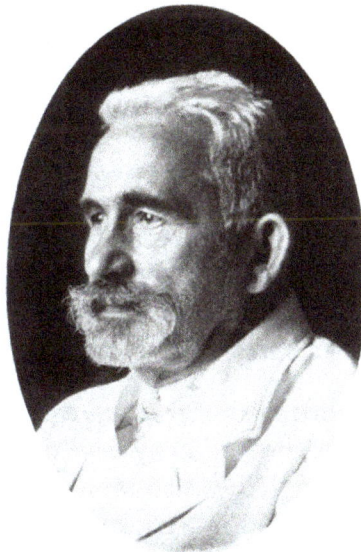

German psychiatrist Emil Kraepelin first distinguished between manic–depressive illness and "dementia praecox" (now known as schizophrenia) in the late 19th century

In the early 1800s, French psychiatrist Jean-Étienne Dominique Esquirol's lypemania, one of his affective monomanias, was the first elaboration on what was to become modern depression. The basis of the current conceptualisation of bipolar illness can be traced back to the 1850s; on January 31, 1854, Jules Baillarger described to the French Imperial Académie Nationale de Médecine a biphasic mental illness causing recurrent oscillations between mania and depression, which he termed *folie à double forme* (dual-form insanity). Two weeks later, on February 14, 1854, Jean-Pierre Falret presented a description to the Academy on what was essentially the same disorder, and which he called *folie circulaire* (circular insanity).

These concepts were developed by the German psychiatrist Emil Kraepelin (1856–1926), who, using Kahlbaum's concept of cyclothymia, categorized and studied the natural course of untreated bipolar patients. He coined the term *manic depressive psychosis*, after noting that periods of acute illness, manic or depressive, were generally punctuated by relatively symptom-free intervals where the patient was able to function normally.

The term "manic–depressive *reaction*" appeared in the first version of the DSM in 1952, influenced by the legacy of Adolf Meyer. Subtyping into "unipolar" depressive disorders and bipolar disorders was first proposed by German psychiatrists Karl Kleist and Karl Leonhard in the 1950s and they have regarded as a separate conditions since publication of the DSM-III. The subtypes bipolar II and rapid cycling have been included since the DSM-IV, based on work from the 1970s by David Dunner, Elliot Gershon, Frederick Goodwin, Ronald Fieve and Joseph Fleiss.

Society and Culture

There are widespread problems with social stigma, stereotypes, and prejudice against individuals with a diagnosis of bipolar disorder.

Kay Redfield Jamison, a clinical psychologist and professor of psychiatry at the Johns Hopkins University School of Medicine, profiled her own bipolar disorder in her memoir *An Unquiet Mind* (1995). In his autobiography *Manicdotes: There's Madness in His Method* (2008) Chris Joseph describes his struggle between the creative dynamism which allowed the creation of his multimillion-pound advertising agency Hook Advertising, and the money-squandering dark despair of his bipolar illness.

Several dramatic works have portrayed characters with traits suggestive of the diagnosis that has been the subject of discussion by psychiatrists and film experts alike. A notable example is *Mr. Jones* (1993), in which Mr. Jones (Richard Gere) swings from a manic episode into a depressive phase and back again, spending time in a psychiatric hospital and displaying many of the features of the syndrome. In *The Mosquito Coast* (1986), Allie Fox (Harrison Ford) displays some features including recklessness, grandiosity, increased goal-directed activity and mood lability, as well as some paranoia. Psychiatrists have suggested that Willy Loman, the main character in Arthur Miller's classic play *Death of a Salesman*, suffers from bipolar disorder, though that specific term for the condition did not exist when the play was written.

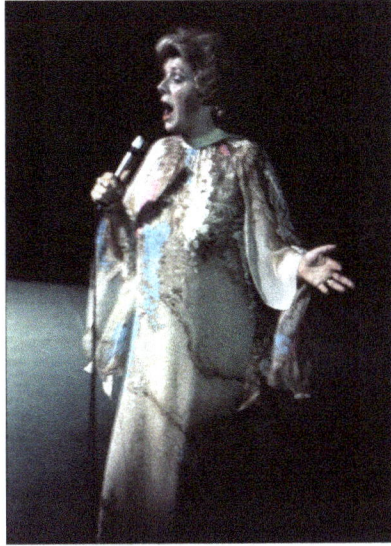

Singer Rosemary Clooney's public revelation of bipolar disorder in 1977 made her an early celebrity spokeswoman for mental illness

TV specials, for example the BBC's *Stephen Fry: The Secret Life of the Manic Depressive*, MTV's *True Life: I'm Bipolar*, talk shows, and public radio shows, and the greater willingness of public figures to discuss their own bipolar disorder, have focused on psychiatric conditions, thereby, raising public awareness.

On April 7, 2009, the nighttime drama *90210* on the CW network, aired a special episode where the character Silver was diagnosed with bipolar disorder. Stacey Slater, a character from the BBC soap EastEnders, has been diagnosed with the disorder. The storyline was developed as part of the BBC's Headroom campaign. The Channel 4 soap *Brookside* had earlier featured a story about bipolar disorder when the character Jimmy Corkhill was diagnosed with the condition. 2011 Showtime's political thriller drama *Homeland* protagonist Carrie Mathison is bipolar, which she has kept secret since her school days. In April 2014, ABC premiered a medical drama, *Black Box*, in which the main character, a world-renowned neuroscientist, is bipolar.

Specific Populations

Children

In the 1920s, Emil Kraepelin noted that manic episodes are rare before puberty. In general, bipolar disorder in children was not recognized in the first half of the twentieth century. This issue diminished with an increased following of the DSM criteria in the last part of the twentieth century.

While in adults the course of bipolar disorder is characterized by discrete episodes of depression and mania with no clear symptomatology between them, in children and adolescents very fast mood changes or even chronic symptoms are the norm. Pediatric bipolar disorder is commonly characterized by outbursts of anger, irritability and psychosis, rather than euphoric mania, which is more likely to be seen in adults. Early onset bipolar disorder is more likely to manifest as depression rather than mania or hypomania.

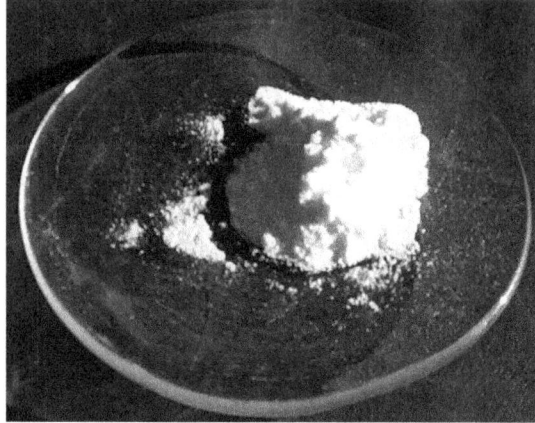

Lithium is the only medication approved by the FDA for treating mania in children

The diagnosis of childhood bipolar disorder is controversial, although it is not under discussion that the typical symptoms of bipolar disorder have negative consequences for minors suffering them. The debate is mainly centered on whether what is called bipolar disorder in children refers to the same disorder as when diagnosing adults, and the related question of whether the criteria for diagnosis for adults are useful and accurate when applied to children. Regarding diagnosis of children, some experts recommend following the DSM criteria. Others believe that these criteria do not correctly separate children with bipolar disorder from other problems such as ADHD, and emphasize fast mood cycles. Still others argue that what accurately differentiates children with bipolar disorder is irritability. The practice parameters of the AACAP encourage the first strategy. American children and adolescents diagnosed with bipolar disorder in community hospitals increased 4-fold reaching rates of up to 40 percent in 10 years around the beginning of the 21st century, while in outpatient clinics it doubled reaching 6 percent. Studies using DSM criteria show that up to 1 percent of youth may have bipolar disorder.

Treatment involves medication and psychotherapy. Drug prescription usually consists in mood stabilizers and atypical antipsychotics. Among the former, lithium is the only compound approved by the FDA for children. Psychological treatment combines normally education on the disease, group therapy and cognitive behavioral therapy. Chronic medication is often needed.

Current research directions for bipolar disorder in children include optimizing treatments, increasing the knowledge of the genetic and neurobiological basis of the pediatric disorder and improving diagnostic criteria. Some treatment research suggests that psychosocial interventions that involve the family, psychoeducation, and skills building (through therapies such as CBT, DBT, and IPSRT) can benefit in a pharmocotherapy. Unfortunately, the literature and research on the effects of psychosocial therapy on BPSD is scarce, making it difficult to determine the efficacy of various therapies. The DSM-5 has proposed a new diagnosis which is considered to cover some presentations currently thought of as childhood-onset bipolar.

Elderly

There is a relative lack of knowledge about bipolar disorder in late life. There is evidence that it becomes less prevalent with age but nevertheless accounts for a similar percentage of psychiatric admissions; that older bipolar patients had first experienced symptoms at a later age; that later onset of mania is associated with more neurologic impairment; that substance abuse is considerably less common in older groups; and that there is probably a greater degree of variation in presentation and course, for instance individuals may develop new-onset mania associated with vascular changes, or become manic only after recurrent depressive episodes, or may have been diagnosed with bipolar disorder at an early age and still meet criteria. There is also some weak and not conclusive evidence that mania is less intense and there is a higher prevalence of mixed episodes, although there may be a reduced response to treatment. Overall, there are likely more similarities than differences from younger adults. In the elderly, recognition and treatment of bipolar disorder may be complicated by the presence of dementia or the side effects of medications being taken for other conditions.

References

- Sethi NK, Robilotti E, Sadan Y (2005). "Neurological Manifestations Of Vitamin B-12 Deficiency". The Internet Journal of Nutrition and Wellness. 2 (1). doi:10.5580/5a9

- Palmer BF, Gates JR, Lader M (2003). "Causes and Management of Hyponatremia". Annals of Pharmacotherapy. 37 (11): 1694–702. PMID 14565794. doi:10.1345/aph.1D105

- Goodman, Brunton L, Chabner B, Knollman B (2011). Goodman Gilman's pharmacological basis of therapeuti (Twelfth ed.). New York: McGraw-Hill Professional. ISBN 978-0-07-162442-8

- Melinda Smith, M.A., Lawrence Robinson, Jeanne Segal, and Damon Ramsey, MD (1 March 2012). "The Bipolar Medication Guide". HelpGuide.org. Retrieved 23 March 2012

- Masalha R, Chudakov B, Muhamad M, Rudoy I, Volkov I, Wirguin I (2001). "Cobalamin-responsive psychosis as the sole manifestation of vitamin B_{12} deficiency". Israeli Medical Association Journal. 3: 701–703

- Behrman, Andy (2002). Electroboy: A Memoir of Mania. Random House Trade Paperbacks. pp. Preface: Flying High. ISBN 978-0-8129-6708-1

- Depression (PDF). National Institute of Mental Health (NIMH). Archived from the original on 27 July 2011. Retrieved 7 September 2008

- Giedke H, Schwärzler F (2002). "Therapeutic use of sleep deprivation in depression". Sleep Medicine Reviews. 6 (5): 361–77. PMID 12531127. doi:10.1053/smrv.2002.0235

- Grant BF (1995). "Comorbidity between DSM-IV drug use disorders and major depression: Results of a national survey of adults". Journal of Substance Abuse. 7 (4): 481–87. PMID 8838629. doi:10.1016/0899-3289(95)90017-9

- "Insomnia: Assessment and Management in Primary Care". American Family Physician. 59 (11): 3029–38. 1999. Retrieved 12 November 2014

- Simon, Gregory E (9 January 2017). "Treating depression in patients with chronic disease". Western Journal of Medicine. 175 (5): 292–293. PMC 1071593. PMID 11694462

- Parker GB, Brotchie H, Graham RK (2017). "Vitamin D and depression". J Affect Disord. 208: 56–61. PMID 27750060. doi:10.1016/j.jad.2016.08.082

- "Depression". National Institute for Health and Care Excellence. December 2004. Archived from the original on 15 November 2008. Retrieved 20 March 2013

- Adell, Albert (1 April 2015). "Revisiting the role of raphe and serotonin in neuropsychiatric disorders". The Journal of General Physiology. 145 (4): 257–259. doi:10.1085/jgp.201511389

- Roth, Anthony; Fonagy, Peter (2005) [1996]. What Works for Whom? Second Edition: A Critical Review of Psychotherapy Research. Guilford Press. p. 78. ISBN 1-59385-272-X

- "Management of depression in primary and secondary care" (PDF). National Clinical Practice Guideline Number 23. National Institute for Health and Clinical Excellence. 2007. Retrieved 4 November 2008

- Krishnadas, Rajeev; Cavanagh, Jonathan (1 May 2012). "Depression: an inflammatory illness?". Journal of Neurology, Neurosurgery, and Psychiatry. 83 (5): 495–502. PMID 22423117. doi:10.1136/jnnp-2011-301779

- Weersing VR, Walker PN (2008). "Review: Cognitive behavioural therapy for adolescents with depression". Evidence-Based Mental Health. 11 (3): 76. PMID 18669678. doi:10.1136/ebmh.11.3.76. Retrieved 27 November 2008

- "Limbic-cortical dysregulation: a proposed model of depression". The Journal of Neuropsychiatry and Clinical Neurosciences. 9 (3): 471–481. 1 August 1997. doi:10.1176/jnp.9.3.471

- Richards, C. Steven; O'Hara, Michael W. (2014). The Oxford Handbook of Depression and Comorbidity. Oxford University Press. p. 254. ISBN 9780199797042

- Hammad TA (16 August 2004). "Review and evaluation of clinical data. Relationship between psychiatric drugs and pediatric suicidality" (PDF). FDA. pp. 42; 115. Retrieved 29 May 2008

- Young RC, Biggs JT, Ziegler VE, Meyer DA (Nov 1978). "A rating scale for mania: reliability, validity and sensitivity". Br J Psychiatry. 133 (5): 429–35. PMID 728692. doi:10.1192/bjp.133.5.429

3

Symptoms of Mood Disorders

Mood disorders can have severe, often crippling symptoms. Some of these which have been listed in this section include hallucination, emotional dysregulation, mood swing, depression and racing thoughts. The topics discussed in the chapter are of great importance to broaden the existing knowledge on mood disorders.

Hallucination

A hallucination is a perception in the absence of external stimulus that has qualities of real perception. Hallucinations are vivid, substantial, and are perceived to be located in external objective space. They are distinguishable from these related phenomena: dreaming, which does not involve wakefulness; illusion, which involves distorted or misinterpreted real perception; imagery, which does not mimic real perception and is under voluntary control; and pseudohallucination, which does not mimic real perception, but is not under voluntary control. Hallucinations also differ from "delusional perceptions", in which a correctly sensed and interpreted stimulus (i.e., a real perception) is given some additional (and typically absurd) significance.

Hallucinations can occur in any sensory modality—visual, auditory, olfactory, gustatory, tactile, proprioceptive, equilibrioceptive, nociceptive, thermoceptive and chronoceptive.

A mild form of hallucination is known as a *disturbance*, and can occur in most of the senses above. These may be things like seeing movement in peripheral vision, or hearing faint noises and/or voices. Auditory hallucinations are very common in schizophrenia. They may be benevolent (telling the subject good things about themselves) or malicious, cursing the subject etc. Auditory hallucinations of the malicious type are frequently heard, for example people talking about the subject behind his/her back. Like auditory hallucinations, the source of the visual counterpart can also be behind the subject's back. Their visual counterpart is the feeling of being looked or stared at, usually with malicious intent. Frequently, auditory hallucinations and their visual counterpart are experienced by the subject together.

Hypnagogic hallucinations and hypnopompic hallucinations are considered normal phenomena. Hypnagogic hallucinations can occur as one is falling asleep and hypnopompic hallucinations occur when one is waking up. Hallucinations can be associated with drug use (particularly deliriants), sleep deprivation, psychosis, neurological disorders, and delirium tremens.

The word "hallucination" itself was introduced into the English language by the 17th century physician Sir Thomas Browne in 1646 from the derivation of the Latin word *alucinari* meaning to wander in the mind. For Browne, hallucination means a sort of vision that is "depraved and receive[s] its objects erroneously".

Classification

Hallucinations may be manifested in a variety of forms. Various forms of hallucinations affect different senses, sometimes occurring simultaneously, creating multiple sensory hallucinations for those experiencing them.

Visual

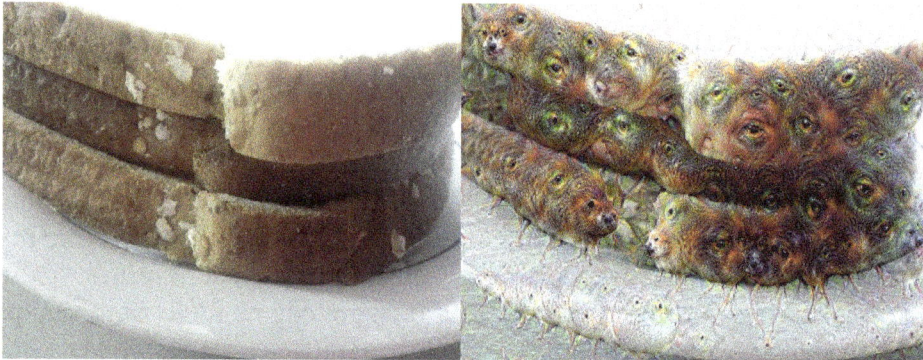

DeepDream modified toast sandwich

A visual hallucination is "the perception of an external visual stimulus where none exists". Alternatively, a visual illusion is a distortion of a real external stimulus. Visual hallucinations are separated into simple and complex.

- Simple visual hallucinations (SVH) are also referred to as non-formed visual hallucinations and elementary visual hallucinations. These terms refer to lights, colors, geometric shapes, and indiscrete objects. These can be further subdivided into phosphenes which are SVH without structure, and photopsias which are SVH with geometric structures.

- Complex visual hallucinations (CVH) are also referred to as formed visual hallucinations. CVHs are clear, lifelike images or scenes such as people, animals, objects, etc.

For example, one may report hallucinating a giraffe. A simple visual hallucination is an amorphous figure that may have a similar shape or color to a giraffe (looks like a giraffe), while a complex visual hallucination is a discrete, lifelike image that is, unmistakably, a giraffe.

Auditory

Auditory hallucinations (also known as *paracusia*) are the perception of sound without outside stimulus. Auditory hallucinations are the most common type of hallucination. Auditory hallucinations can be divided into two categories: elementary and complex. Elementary hallucinations are the perception of sounds such as hissing, whistling, an extended tone, and more. In many cases, tinnitus is an elementary auditory hallucination. However, some people who experience certain types of tinnitus, especially pulsatile tinnitus, are actually hearing the blood rushing through vessels near the ear. Because the auditory stimulus is present in this situation, it does not qualify as a hallucination.

Complex hallucinations are those of voices, music, or other sounds that may or may not be clear, may be familiar or completely unfamiliar, and friendly or aggressive, among other possibilities. A hallucination of a single individual person of one or more talking voices are particularly associated with psychotic disorders such as schizophrenia, and hold special significance in diagnosing these conditions.

If a group of people experience a complex auditory hallucination, no single individual can be named psychotic or schizophrenic.

Another typical disorder where auditory hallucinations are very common is dissociative identity disorder. In schizophrenia voices are normally perceived coming from outside the person but in dissociative disorders they are perceived as originating from within the person, commenting in their head not behind their back. Differential diagnosis between schizophrenia and dissociative disorders is challenging due to many overlapping symptoms especially Schneiderian first rank symptoms such as hallucinations. However, many people not suffering from diagnosable mental illness may sometimes hear voices as well. One important example to consider when forming a differential diagnosis for a patient with paracusia is lateral temporal lobe epilepsy. Despite the tendency to associate hearing voices, or otherwise hallucinating, and psychosis with schizophrenia or other psychiatric illnesses, it is crucial to take into consideration that, even if a person does exhibit psychotic features, he/she does not necessarily suffer from a psychiatric disorder on its own. Disorders such as Wilson's disease, various endocrine diseases, numerous metabolic disturbances, multiple sclerosis, systemic lupus erythematosus, porphyria, sarcoidosis, and many others can present with psychosis.

Musical hallucinations are also relatively common in terms of complex auditory hallucinations and may be the result of a wide range of causes ranging from hearing-loss (such as in musical ear syndrome, the auditory version of Charles Bonnet syndrome), lateral temporal lobe epilepsy, arteriovenous malformation, stroke, lesion, abscess, or tumor.

The Hearing Voices Movement is a support and advocacy group for people who hallucinate voices, but do not otherwise show signs of mental illness or impairment.

High caffeine consumption has been linked to an increase in the likelihood of one's experiencing auditory hallucinations. A study conducted by the La Trobe University School of Psychological Sciences revealed that as few as five cups of coffee a day (approximately 500 mg of caffeine) could trigger the phenomenon.

Command

Command hallucinations are hallucinations in the form of commands; they can be auditory or inside of the person's mind and/or consciousness. The contents of the hallucinations can range from the innocuous to commands to cause harm to the self or others. Command hallucinations are often associated with schizophrenia. People experiencing command hallucinations may or may not comply with the hallucinated commands, depending on the circumstances. Compliance is more common for non-violent commands.

Command hallucinations are sometimes used in defense of a crime, often homicides. In essence, it is a voice that one hears and it tells the listener what to do. Sometimes the commands are quite benign directives such as "Stand up" or "Shut the door." Whether it is a command for something simple or something that is a threat, it is still considered a "command hallucination." Some helpful questions that can assist one in figuring out if he/she may be suffering from this include: "What are the voices telling you to do?", "When did your voices first start telling you to do things?", "Do you recognize the person who is telling you to harm yourself (or others)?", "Do you think you can resist doing what the voices are telling you to do?"

Olfactory

Phantosmia (olfactory hallucinations), smelling an odor that is not actually there, and parosmia (olfactory illusions), inhaling a real odor but perceiving it as different scent than remembered, are distortions to the sense of smell (olfactory system) that, in most cases, are not caused by anything serious and usually go away on their own in time. It can result from a range of conditions such as nasal infections, nasal polyps, dental problems, migraines, head injuries, seizures, strokes, or brain tumors. Environmental exposures are sometimes the cause as well, such as smoking, exposure to certain types of chemicals (e.g., insecticides or solvents), or radiation treatment for head or neck cancer. It can also be a symptom of certain mental disorders such as depression, bipolar disorder, intoxication or withdrawal from drugs and alcohol, or psychotic disorders (e.g., schizophrenia). The perceived odors are usually unpleasant and commonly described as smelling burned, foul spoiled, or rotten.

Tactile

Tactile hallucinations are the illusion of tactile sensory input, simulating various types of pressure to the skin or other organs. One subtype of tactile hallucination, formication, is the sensation of insects crawling underneath the skin and is frequently associated with prolonged cocaine use. However, formication may also be the result of normal hormonal changes such as menopause, or disorders such as peripheral neuropathy, high fevers, Lyme disease, skin cancer, and more.

Gustatory

This type of hallucination is the perception of taste without a stimulus. These hallucinations, which are typically strange or unpleasant, are relatively common among individuals who have certain types of focal epilepsy, especially temporal lobe epilepsy. The regions of the brain responsible for gustatory hallucination in this case are the insula and the superior bank of the sylvian fissure.

General somatic Sensations

General somatic sensations of a hallucinatory nature are experienced when an individual feels that their body is being mutilated, i.e. twisted, torn, or disembowelled. Other reported cases are invasion by animals in the person's internal organs such as snakes in the stomach or frogs in the rectum. The general feeling that one's flesh is decomposing is also classified under this type of hallucination.

Cause

Hallucinations can be caused by a number of factors.

Hypnagogic Hallucination

These hallucinations occur just before falling asleep, and affect a high proportion of the population: in one survey 37% of the respondents experienced them twice a week. The hallucinations can last from seconds to minutes; all the while, the subject usually remains aware of the true nature of the images. These may be associated with narcolepsy. Hypnagogic hallucinations are sometimes associated with brainstem abnormalities, but this is rare.

Peduncular Hallucinosis

Peduncular means pertaining to the peduncle, which is a neural tract running to and from the pons on the brain stem. These hallucinations usually occur in the evenings, but not during drowsiness, as in the case of hypnagogic hallucination. The subject is usually fully conscious and then can interact with the hallucinatory characters for extended periods of time. As in the case of hypnagogic hallucinations, insight into the nature of the images remains intact. The false images can occur in any part of the visual field, and are rarely polymodal.

Delirium Tremens

One of the more enigmatic forms of visual hallucination is the highly variable, possibly polymodal delirium tremens. Individuals suffering from delirium tremens may be agitated and confused, especially in the later stages of this disease. Insight is gradually reduced with the progression of this disorder. Sleep is disturbed and occurs for a shorter period of time, with rapid eye movement sleep.

Parkinson's Disease and Lewy Body Dementia

Parkinson's disease is linked with Lewy body dementia for their similar hallucinatory symptoms. The symptoms strike during the evening in any part of the visual field, and are rarely polymodal. The segue into hallucination may begin with illusions where sensory perception is greatly distorted, but no novel sensory information is present. These typically last for several minutes, during which time the subject may be either conscious and normal or drowsy/inaccessible. Insight into these hallucinations is usually preserved and REM sleep is usually reduced. Parkinson's disease is usually associated with a degraded substantia nigra pars compacta, but recent evidence suggests that PD affects a number of sites in the brain. Some places of noted degradation include the median raphe nuclei, the noradrenergic parts of the locus coeruleus, and the cholinergic neurons in the parabrachial area and pedunculopontine nuclei of the tegmentum.

Migraine Coma

This type of hallucination is usually experienced during the recovery from a comatose state. The migraine coma can last for up to two days, and a state of depression is sometimes comorbid. The hallucinations occur during states of full consciousness, and insight into the hallucinatory nature of the images is preserved. It has been noted that ataxic lesions accompany the migraine coma.

Charles Bonnet Syndrome

Charles Bonnet syndrome is the name given to visual hallucinations experienced by a partially or severely sight impaired person. The hallucinations can occur at any time and can distress people of any age, as they may not initially be aware that they are hallucinating, they may fear initially for their own mental health which may delay them sharing with carers what is happening until they start to understand it themselves. The hallucinations can frighten and disconcert as to what is real and what is not and carers need to learn how to support sufferers. The hallucinations can sometimes be dispersed by eye movements, or perhaps just reasoned logic such as, "I can see fire but there is no smoke and there is no heat from it" or perhaps "We have an infestation of rats but they have pink ribbons with a bell tied on their necks." Over elapsed months and years the manifestation of the hallucinations may change, becoming more or less frequent with changes in ability to see. The length of time that the sight impaired person can suffer from these hallucinations varies according to the underlying speed of eye deterioration. A differential diagnosis are ophthalmopathic hallucinations.

Focal Epilepsy

Visual hallucinations due to focal seizures differ depending on the region of the brain where the seizure occurs. For example, visual hallucinations during occipital lobe seizures are typically visions of brightly colored, geometric shapes that may move across the visual field, multiply, or form concentric rings and generally persist from a few seconds to a few minutes. They are usually unilateral and localized to one part of the visual field on the contralateral side of the seizure focus, typically the temporal field. However, unilateral visions moving horizontally across the visual field begin on the contralateral side and move toward the ipsilateral side.

Temporal lobe seizures, on the other hand, can produce complex visual hallucinations of people, scenes, animals, and more as well as distortions of visual perception. Complex hallucinations may appear real or unreal, may or may not be distorted with respect to size, and may seem disturbing or affable, among other variables. One rare but notable type of hallucination is heautoscopy, a hallucination of a mirror image of one's self. These "other selves" may be perfectly still or performing complex tasks, may be an image of a younger self or the present self, and tend to be only briefly present. Complex hallucinations are a relatively uncommon finding in temporal lobe epilepsy patients. Rarely, they may occur during occipital focal seizures or in parietal lobe seizures.

Distortions in visual perception during a temporal lobe seizure may include size distortion (micropsia or macropsia), distorted perception of movement (where moving objects may appear to be moving very slowly or to be perfectly still), a sense that surfaces such as ceilings and even entire horizons are moving farther away in a fashion similar to the dolly zoom effect, and other illusions. Even when consciousness is impaired, insight into the hallucination or illusion is typically preserved.

Drug-induced Hallucination

Drug-induced hallucinations are caused by the consumption of psychoactive substances such as deliriants, psychedelics, and certain stimulants, which are known to cause visual and auditory hallucinations. Some psychedelics such as lysergic acid diethylamide and psilocybin can cause hallucinations that range from a spectrum of mild to severe. Some of these drugs can be used in psychotherapy to treat mental disorders, addiction, anxiety, and secondary to advanced stage cancers.

Sensory Deprivation Hallucination

Hallucinations can be caused by sense deprivation when it occurs for prolonged periods of time, and almost always occur in the modality being deprived (visual for blindfolded/darkness, auditory for muffled conditions, etc.)

Experimentally-induced Hallucinations

Anomalous experiences, such as so-called benign hallucinations, may occur in a person in a state of good mental and physical health, even in the apparent absence of a transient trigger factor such as fatigue, intoxication or sensory deprivation. It is now widely recognized that hallucinatory experiences are not merely the prerogative of those suffering from mental illness, or normal people in abnormal states, but that they occur spontaneously in a significant proportion of the normal population, when in good health and not undergoing particular stress or other abnormal circumstance.

The evidence for this statement has been accumulating for more than a century. Studies of benign hallucinatory experiences go back to 1886 and the early work of the Society for Psychical Research, which suggested approximately 10% of the population had experienced at least one hallucinatory episode in the course of their life. More recent studies have validated these findings; the precise incidence found varies with the nature of the episode and the criteria of 'hallucination' adopted, but the basic finding is now well-supported.

Non-celiac Gluten Sensitivity

Non-celiac gluten sensitivity can cause hallucinations in some people, which some authors have termed "gluten psychosis".

Pathophysiology

Visual

Sometimes internal imagery can overwhelm the sensory input from external stimuli when sharing neural pathways, or if indistinct stimuli is perceived and manipulated to match one's expectations or beliefs, especially about the environment. This can result in a hallucination, and this effect is sometimes exploited to form an optical illusion.

There are three pathophysiologic mechanisms thought to account for complex visual hallucinations. These mechanisms consist of the following:

- Irritation of cortical centers responsible for visual processing (e.g., seizure activity). The irritation of the primary visual cortex causes simple elementary visual hallucinations.

- Lesions that cause deafferentation of the visual system may lead to cortical release phenomenon, which includes visual hallucination.

- The reticular activating system, which has been linked to the genesis of visual hallucinations.

Some specific classifications include: elementary hallucinations, which may entail flicks, specks, and bars of light (called phosphenes). Closed eye hallucinations in darkness, which are common to psychedelic drugs (i.e., LSD, mescaline). Scenic or "panoramic" hallucinations, which are not superimposed but vividly replace the entire visual field with hallucinatory content similarly to dreams; such scenic hallucinations may occur in epilepsy (in which they are usually stereotyped and experimental in character), hallucinogen use, and more rarely in catatonic schizophrenia (cf. oneirophrenia), mania, and brainstem lesions, among others.

Another thing that may cause visual hallucinations is prolonged visual deprivation. In a study where 13 healthy people were blindfolded for 5 days, 10 out of the 13 subjects reported visual hallucinations. This finding lends strong support to the idea that the simple loss of normal visual input is sufficient to cause visual hallucinations.

Psychodynamic View

Various theories have been put forward to explain the occurrence of hallucinations. When psychodynamic (Freudian) theories were popular in psychology, hallucinations were seen as a projection of unconscious wishes, thoughts, and wants. As biological theories have become orthodox, hallucinations are more often thought of (by psychologists at least) as being caused by functional deficits in the brain. With reference to mental illness, the function (or dysfunction) of the neurotransmitters glutamate and dopamine are thought to be particularly important. The Freudian interpretation may have an aspect of truth, as the biological hypothesis explains the physical interactions in the brain, while the Freudian interpretation addresses the psychological complexes related to the content of the hallucination, such as hallucinating persecutory voices due to guilt. Psychological research has argued that hallucinations may result from biases in what are known as metacognitive abilities.

Information Processing Perspective

These are abilities that allow us to monitor or draw inferences from our own internal psychological states (such as intentions, memories, beliefs and thoughts). The ability to discriminate between internal (self-generated) and external (stimuli) sources of information is considered to be an important metacognitive skill, but one which may break down to cause hallucinatory experiences. Projection of an internal state (or a person's own reaction to another's) may arise in the form of hallucinations, especially auditory hallucinations. A recent hypothesis that is gaining acceptance concerns the role of overactive top-down processing, or strong perceptual expectations, that can generate spontaneous perceptual output (that is, hallucination).

Stages of Hallucination

1. Emergence of surprising or warded-off memory or fantasy images

2. Frequent reality checks

3. Last vestige of insight as hallucinations become indistinguishable from reality.

4. Fantasy and distortion elaborated upon and confused with actual perception

5. Internal-external boundaries destroyed and possible pantheistic (or personally felt or believed, possibly profound, internal spiritual or religious) experience

Biological Perspective

Auditory Hallucinations

Auditory hallucinations are the most prevalent type of hallucinations. They include hearing voices and music. Many times an individual suffering from auditory hallucinations will hear a voice or voices saying the individual's own thoughts out loud, commenting on all their actions, or commanding and ordering the individual around. These voices tend to be negative and critical toward the individual. People who suffer from schizophrenia and have auditory hallucinations will often speak to the voice as though they are speaking to a second person.

Visual

The most common modality referred to when people speak of hallucinations include the phenomena of seeing things that are not present or visual perception, which does not reconcile with the physical, consensus reality. There are many different causes that have been classed as psychophysiologic (a disturbance of brain structure), psychobiochemical (a disturbance of neurotransmitters), psychodynamic (an emergence of the unconscious into consciousness), and psychological (e.g., meaningful experiences consciousness); this is also the case in Alzheimer's disease. Numerous disorders can involve visual hallucinations, ranging from psychotic disorders to dementia to migraine, but experiencing visual hallucinations does not in itself mean that there is necessarily a disorder. Visual hallucinations are associated with organic disorders of the brain and with drug- and alcohol-related illness, and not typically considered the result of a psychiatric disorder.

Schizoc Hallucination

Hallucinations may be caused by schizophrenia. Schizophrenia is a mental disorder in which there is an inability to tell the difference between real and unreal experiences, to think logically, to have contextually appropriate emotions, and to function in social situations.

Neuroanatomical Correlates

Normal everyday procedures like getting an MRI (Magnetic Resonance Imaging) have been used to find out more about auditory and verbal hallucinations. "Functional magnetic resonance imaging (fMRI) and repetitive transcranial magnetic stimulation (rTMS) were used to explore the pathophysiology of auditory/verbal hallucinations (AVHs)" Throughout the exploring through MRI's of patients, there were "lower levels of hallucination-related activation in Broca's area strongly predicted greater rate of response to left temporoparietal rTMS."

Also through fMRIs, it is found that there can be better understandings on why hallucinations happen in the brain, by understanding emotions and cognition and how they can prompt physical reactions that can help result in a hallucination. It suggests the theory that "motivations in the body and mind can drive us to certain behaviors that we act in, such as survival instinct and intuition" and that they can work in a hand-in-hand-like fashion. It can also be viewed as a symbolic "homeostasis" that can have adverse effects by having these hallucinations and/or mental illnesses. The amygdala has also been seen to relate to this finding by contributing a "declarative judgement of emotional salience" as well as affecting both "efferent and afferent representational levels of affective autonomic responses in the brain". Hallucinations in schizophrenia have been found to associate with differences in morphology of the paracingulate sulcus.

Pathophysiological Mechanisms

There are symptoms that are mechanism-based that are associated with hallucinations. These include superficial pressure and stabbing pain. Others include a burning-like sensation or electric shock feeling. Human studies of these symptoms remain mostly unclear unlike similar studies in animals.

Treatments

There are few treatments for many types of hallucinations. However, for those hallucinations caused by mental disease, a psychologist or psychiatrist should be alerted, and treatment will be based on the observations of those doctors. Antipsychotic and atypical antipsychotic medication may also be utilized to treat the illness if the symptoms are severe and cause significant distress. For other causes of hallucinations there is no factual evidence to support any one treatment is scientifically tested and proven. However, abstaining from hallucinogenic drugs, managing stress levels, living healthily, and getting plenty of sleep can help reduce the prevalence of hallucinations. In all cases of hallucinations, medical attention should be sought out and informed of one's specific symptoms.

Epidemiology

One study from as early as 1895 reported that approximately 10% of the population experiences hallucinations. A 1996-1999 survey of over 13,000 people reported a much higher figure, with almost 39% of people reporting hallucinatory experiences, 27% of which daytime hallucinations, mostly outside the context of illness or drug use. From this survey, olfactory (smell) and gustatory (taste) hallucinations seem the most common in the general population.

Emotional Dysregulation

Emotional dysregulation (ED) is a term used in the mental health community to refer to an emotional response that is poorly modulated, and does not fall within the conventionally accepted range of emotive response. ED may be referred to as labile mood (marked fluctuation of mood) or mood swings.

Possible manifestations of emotional dysregulation include angry outbursts or behavior outbursts such as destroying or throwing objects, aggression towards self or others, and threats to kill oneself. These variations usually occur in seconds to minutes or hours. Emotional dysregulation can lead to behavioral problems and can interfere with a person's social interactions and relationships at home, in school, or at place of employment.

Emotional dysregulation can be associated with an experience of early psychological trauma, brain injury, or chronic maltreatment (such as child abuse, child neglect, or institutional neglect/abuse), and associated disorders such as reactive attachment disorder. Emotional dysregulation may present in people with psychiatric disorders such as attention deficit hyperactivity disorder, bipolar disorder, borderline personality disorder, and complex post-traumatic stress disorder. ED is also found among those with autism spectrum disorders, including Asperger syndrome. In such cases as borderline personality disorder, hypersensitivity to emotional stimuli causes a slower return to a normal emotional state. This is manifested biologically by deficits in the frontal cortices of the brain.

Etymology

The word "dysregulation" is a neologism created by combining the prefix "dys-" to "regulation". According to *Webster's Dictionary*, dys- has various roots. With Latin and Greek roots, it is akin to Old English *tō-*, *te-* "apart" and in Sanskrit *dus-*" bad, difficult."

Child Psychopathology

There are links between child emotional dysregulation and later psychopathology. For instance, ADHD symptoms are associated with problems with emotional regulation, motivation, and arousal. One study found a connection between emotional dysregulation at 5 and 10 months, and parent-reported problems with anger and distress at 18 months. Low levels of emotional regulation behaviors at 5 months were also related to non-compliant behaviors at 30 months. While links have been found between emotional dysregulation and child psychopathology, the mechanisms behind how early emotional dysregulation and later psychopathology are related are not yet clear.

Symptoms

Smoking, self-harm, eating disorders, and addiction have all been associated with emotional dysregulation. Somatoform disorders may be caused by a decreased ability to regulate and experience emotions or an inability to express emotions in a positive way. Individuals who have difficulty regulating emotions are at risk for eating disorders and substance abuse as they use food or substances as a way to regulate their emotions. Emotional dysregulation is also found in people who are at increased risk to develop a mental disorder, in particular an affective disorder such as depression or bipolar disorder.

Early Childhood

Research has shown that failures in emotional regulation may be related to the display of acting out, externalizing disorders, or behavior problems. When presented with challenging tasks, children who were found to have defects in emotional regulation (high-risk) spent less time attending to tasks and more time throwing tantrums or fretting than children without emotional regulation problems (low-risk). These high-risk children had difficulty with self-regulation and had difficulty complying with requests from caregivers and were more defiant. Emotional dysregulation has also been associated with childhood social withdrawal. Common signs of emotional dysregulation in early childhood include isolation, throwing things, screaming, lack of eye contact, refusing to speak, rocking, running away, crying, dissociating, high levels of anxiety, or inability to be flexible.

Internalizing Behaviors

Emotional dysregulation in children can be associated with internalizing behaviors including

- exhibiting emotions too intense for a situation
- difficulty calming down when upset
- difficulty decreasing negative emotions
- being less able to calm themselves
- difficulty understanding emotional experiences
- becoming avoidant or aggressive when dealing with negative emotions
- experiencing more negative emotions

Externalizing Behaviors

Emotional dysregulation in children can be associated with externalizing behaviors including

- exhibiting more extreme emotions
- difficulty identifying emotional cues
- difficulty recognizing their own emotions

- focusing on the negative

- difficulty controlling their attention

- being impulsive

- difficulty decreasing their negative emotions

- difficulty calming down when upset

Protective Factors

Early experiences with caregivers can lead to differences in emotional regulation. The responsiveness of a caregiver to an infant's signals can help an infant regulate their emotional systems. Caregiver interaction styles that overwhelm a child or that are unpredictable may undermine emotional regulation development. Effective strategies involve working with a child to support developing self-control such as modeling a desired behavior rather than demanding it.

The richness of environment that a child is exposed to helps development of emotional regulation. An environment must provide appropriate levels of freedom and constraint. The environment must allow opportunities for a child to practice self-regulation. An environment with opportunities to practice social skills without over-stimulation or excessive frustration helps a child develop self-regulation skills.

Mood Swing

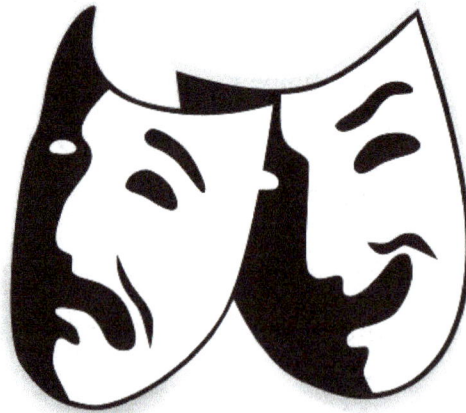

Bipolar disorder is characterized by extreme mood swings, usually between mania and depression

A mood swing is an extreme or rapid change in mood. Such mood swings can play a positive part in promoting problem solving and in producing flexible forward planning.

However, when mood swings are so strong that they are disruptive, they may be the main part of a bipolar disorder.

Overview

Speed and Extent

Mood swings can happen any time at any place, varying from the microscopic to the wild oscillations of manic depression, so that a continuum can be traced from normal struggles around self-esteem, through cyclothymia, up to a depressive disease. However most people's mood swings remain in the mild to moderate range of emotional ups and downs.

The duration of mood swings also varies. They may last a few hours - *ultrarapid* - or extend over days - *ultradian*: clinicians maintain that only when four continuous days of hypomania, or seven days of mania, occur, is a diagnosis of bipolar disorder justified.

In such cases, mood swings can extend over several days, even weeks: these episodes may consist of rapid alternation between feelings of depression and euphoria.

Causes

Changes in a person's energy level, sleep patterns, self-esteem, concentration, drug or alcohol use can be signs of an oncoming mood disorder.

Many different things might trigger mood swings, from unhealthy diet or lifestyle to drug abuse or hormonal imbalance.

Other major causes of mood swings (besides bi-polar disorder and major depression) include diseases/disorders which interfere with nervous system function. Attention deficit hyperactivity disorder (ADHD), epilepsy, and autism are three such examples.

The hyperactivity sometimes accompanied by inattentiveness, impulsiveness, and forgetfulness are cardinal symptoms associated with ADHD. As a result, ADHD is known to bring about usually short-lived (though sometimes dramatic) mood swings. The communication difficulties associated with autism, and the associated changes in neurochemistry, are also known to cause autistic fits (autistic mood swings). The seizures associated with epilepsy involve changes in the brain's electrical firing, and thus may also bring about striking and dramatic mood swings. If the mood swing is not associated with a mood disorder, treatments are harder to assign. Most commonly, however, mood swings are the result of dealing with stressful and/or unexpected situations in daily life.

Degenerative diseases of the human central nervous system such as Parkinson's disease, Alzheimer's disease, multiple sclerosis, and Huntington's disease may also produce mood swings.

Not eating on time can contribute, or eating too much sugar, can cause fluctuations in blood sugar, which can cause mood swings.

Brain Chemistry

If a person has an abnormal level of one or several of certain neurotransmitters (NTs) in their brain, it may result in having mood swings or a mood disorder. Serotonin is one such neurotransmitter that is involved with sleep, moods, and emotional states. A slight imbalance of this NT could result in depression. Norepinephrine is a neurotransmitter that is involved with learning, memory, and physical arousal. Like serotonin, an imbalance of norepinephrine may also result in depression.

List of Conditions known to Cause Mood Swings

- Anabolic steroid abuse
- Attention deficit hyperactivity disorder
- Autism or other pervasive developmental disorder
- Bipolar disorder or cyclothymia
- Borderline personality disorder
- Dementia, including Alzheimer's disease, Parkinson's disease and Huntington's disease
- Epilepsy
- Hypothyroidism or hyperthyroidism
- Intermittent explosive disorder
- Major depression
- Post traumatic stress disorder
- Premenstrual syndrome
- Schizoaffective disorder
- Schizophrenia
- Seasonal affective disorder
- XXYY syndrome

Treatment

Cognitive behavioral therapy recommends using *emotional dampeners* to break the self-reinforcing tendencies of either manic or depressive mood swings. Exercise, treats, seeking out small (and easily attainable) triumphs, and using vicarious distractions like reading or watching TV, are among the techniques found to be regularly used by people in breaking depressive swings.

Learning to bring oneself *down* from grandiose states of mind, or *up* from exaggerated shame states, is part of taking a proactive approach to managing one's own moods and varying sense of self-esteem.

Depression (Differential Diagnoses)

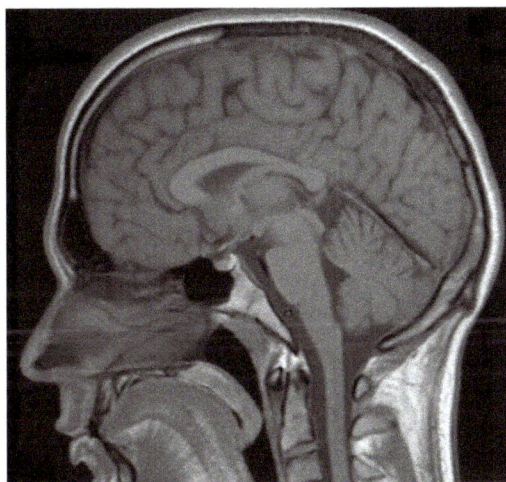

Neuroimaging can be a valuable tool in the diagnostic work-up of various psychiatric disorders including depression.

Depression, one of the most commonly diagnosed psychiatric disorders, is being diagnosed in increasing numbers in various segments of the population worldwide. Depression in the United States alone affects 17.6 million Americans each year or 1 in 6 people. Depressed patients are at increased risk of type 2 diabetes, cardiovascular disease and suicide. Within the next twenty years depression is expected to become the second leading cause of disability worldwide and the leading cause in high-income nations, including the United States. In approximately 75% of completed suicides, the individuals had seen a physician within the prior year before their death, 45–66% within the prior month. About a third of those who completed suicide had contact with mental health services in the prior year, a fifth within the preceding month.

There are many psychiatric and medical conditions that may mimic some or all of the symptoms of depression or may occur comorbid to it. A disorder either psychiatric or medical that shares symptoms and characteristics of another disorder, and may be the true cause of the presenting symptoms is known as a differential diagnosis.

Many psychiatric disorders such as depression are diagnosed by allied health professionals with little or no medical training, and are made on the basis of presenting symptoms without proper consideration of the underlying cause, adequate screening of differential diagnoses is often not conducted. According to one study, "non-medical mental health care providers may be at increased risk of not recognizing masked medical illnesses in their patients."

Misdiagnosis or missed diagnoses may lead to lack of treatment or ineffective and potentially harmful treatment which may worsen the underlying causative disorder. A conservative estimate is that 10% of all psychological symptoms may be due to medical reasons, with the results of one study suggesting that about half of individuals with a serious mental illness "have general medical conditions that are largely undiagnosed and untreated and may cause or exacerbate psychiatric symptoms".

In a case of misdiagnosed depression recounted in *Newsweek*, a writer received treatment for depression for years; during the last 10 years of her depression the symptoms worsened, resulting in multiple suicide attempts and psychiatric hospitalizations. When an MRI finally was performed, it showed the presence of a tumor. However, she was told by a neurologist that it was benign. After a worsening of symptoms, and upon the second opinion of another neurologist, the tumor was removed. After the surgery, she no longer suffered from depressive symptoms.

Autoimmune Disorders

- Celiac disease; is an autoimmune disorder in which the body is unable to digest gluten which is found in various food grains, most notably wheat, and also rye and barley. Current research has shown its neuropsychiatric symptoms may manifest without the gastrointestinal symptoms.

- "However, more recent studies have emphasized that a wider spectrum of neurologic syndromes may be the presenting extraintestinal manifestation of gluten sensitivity with or without intestinal pathology."

- Lupus: Systemic lupus erythematosus (SLE), is a chronic autoimmune connective tissue disease that can affect any part of the body. Lupus can cause or worsen depression.

Bacterial-viral-parasitic Infection

- Lyme disease; is a bacterial infection caused by Borrelia burgdorferi, a spirochete bacterium transmitted by the Deer tick (Ixodes scapularis). Lyme disease is one of a group of diseases which have earned the name the "great imitator" for their propensity to mimic the symptoms of a wide variety of medical and neuropsychiatric disorders. Lyme disease is an underdiagnosed illness, partially as a result of the complexity and unreliability of serologic testing.

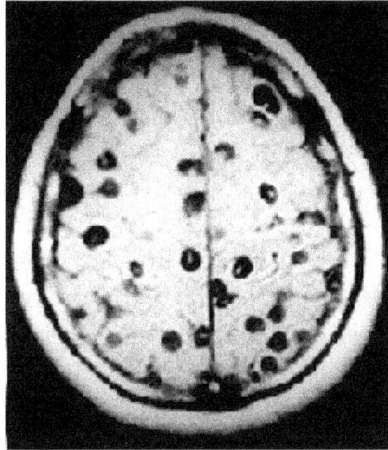
MRI brain scan: Neurocysticercosis

- "Because of the rapid rise of Lyme borreliosis nationwide and the need for antibiotic treatment to prevent severe neurologic damage, mental health professionals need to be aware of its possible psychiatric presentations.

- Syphilis; the prevalence of which is on the rise, is another of the "great imitators", which if left untreated can progress to neurosyphilis and affect the brain, can present with solely neuropsychiatric symptoms. "This case emphasises that neurosyphilis still has to be considered in the differential diagnosis within the context of psychiatric conditions and diseases. Owing to current epidemiological data and difficulties in diagnosing syphilis, routine screening tests in the psychiatric field are necessary."

- Neurocysticercosis (NCC): is an infection of the brain or spinal cord caused by the larval stage of the pork tapeworm, *Taenia solium*. NCC is the most common helminthic (parasitic worm) infestation of the central nervous system worldwide. Humans develop cysticercosis when they ingest eggs of the pork tapeworm via contact with contaminated fecal matter or eating infected vegetables or undercooked pork. "While cysticercosis is endemic in Latin America, it is an emerging disease with increased prevalence in the United States." "The rate of depression in those with neurocysticercosis is higher than in the general population."

- Toxoplasmosis; is an infection caused by *Toxoplasma gondii* an intracellular protozoan parasite. Humans can be infected in 3 different ways: ingestion of tissue cysts, ingestion of oocysts, or in utero infection with tachyzoites. One of the prime methods for transmission to humans is contact with the feces of the host species, the domesticated cat. Toxoplasma gondii infects approximately 30% of the world's human population, but causes overt clinical symptoms in only a small segment of those infected. Exposure to Toxoplasma gondii (seropositivity) without developing Toxoplasmosis has been proven to alter various characteristics of human behavior as well as being a causative factor in some cases of depression, in addition, studies have linked seropositivity with an increased rate of suicide

- West Nile virus (WNV); which can cause encephalitis has been reported to be a causal factor in developing depression in 31% of those infected in a study conducted in Houston, Texas and reported to the Center for Disease Control (CDC). The primary vectors for disease transmission to humans are various species of mosquito. WNV which is endemic to Southern Europe, Africa the Middle East and Asia was first identified in the United States in 1999. Between 1999 and 2006, 20,000 cases of confirmed symptomatic WNV were reported in the United States, with estimates of up to 1 million being infected. "WNV is now the most common cause of epidemic viral encephalitis in the United States, and it will likely remain an important cause of neurological disease for the foreseeable future."

Blood disorders

Anemia: is a decrease in normal number of red blood cells (RBCs) or less than the normal quantity of hemoglobin in the blood. Depressive symptoms are associated with anemia in a general population of older persons living in the community.

Chronic Fatigue Syndrome

Between 1 and 4 million Americans are believed to have Chronic Fatigue Syndrome (CFS), yet only 50% have consulted a physician for symptoms of CFS. In addition individuals with CFS symptoms often have an undiagnosed medical or psychiatric disorder such as diabetes, thyroid disease or substance abuse. CFS, at one time considered to be psychosomatic in nature, is now considered to be a valid medical condition in which early diagnosis and treatment can aid in alleviating or completely resolving symptoms. While frequently misdiagnosed as depression, differences have been noted in rate of cerebral blood flow.

CFS is underdiagnosed in more than 80% of the people who have it; at the same time, it is often misdiagnosed as depression.

Dietary Disorders

- Fructose malabsorption and lactose intolerance; deficient fructose transport by the duodenum, or by the deficiency of the enzyme, lactase in the mucosal lining, respectively. As a result of this malabsorption the saccharides reach the colon and are digested by bacteria which convert them to short chain fatty acids, CO_2, and H_2. Approximately 50% of those afflicted exhibit the physical signs of irritable bowel syndrome.

- "Fructose malabsorption may play a role in the development of depressed mood. Fructose malabsorption should be considered in patients with symptoms of major depression"

- "Fructose and sorbitol reduced diet in subjects with fructose malabsorption does not only reduce gastrointestinal symptoms but also improves mood and early signs of depression."

Endocrine System Disorders

Dysregulation of the endocrine system may present with various neuropsychiatric symptoms; irregularities in the hypothalamic-pituitary- adrenal (HPA) axis and the hypothalamic-pituitary-thyroid (HPT) axis have been shown in patients with primary depression.

HPT and HPA axes abnormalities observed in patients with depression
(Musselman DL, Nemeroff CB. 1996)
HPT axes irregularities:
• alterations in thyroid-stimulating hormone (TSH) response to thyrotropin-releasing hormone (TRH)
• an abnormally high rate of antithyroid antibodies
• elevated cerebrospinal fluid (CSF) TRH concentrations.
HPA axes irregularities:
• adrenocorticoid hypersecretion
• enlarged pituitary and adrenal gland size (organomegaly)
• elevated corticotropin-releasing factor (CSF) concentrations

Adrenal Gland

- Addison's disease: also known as chronic adrenal insufficiency, hypocortisolism, and hypocorticism) is a rare endocrine disorder wherein the adrenal glands, located above the kidneys, produce insufficient steroid hormones (glucocorticoids and often mineralocorticoids). "Addison's disease presenting with psychiatric features in the early stage has the tendency to be overlooked and misdiagnosed."

- Cushing's Syndrome, also known as hypercortisolism, is an endocrine disorder characterized by an excess of cortisol. In the absence of prescribed steroid medications, it is caused by a tumor on the pituitary or adrenal glands, or more rarely, an ectopic hormone-secreting tumor. Depression is a common feature in diagnosed patients and it often improves with treatment.

Thyroid and Parathyroid Glands

- Graves' disease: an autoimmune disease where the thyroid is overactive, resulting in hyperthyroidism and thyrotoxicosis.

- Hashimoto's thyroiditis: also known chronic lymphocytic thyroiditis is an auto-immune disease in which the thyroid gland is gradually destroyed by a variety of cell and antibody mediated immune processes. Hashimoto's thyroiditis is associated with thyroid peroxidase and thyroglobulin autoantibodies

- Hashitoxicosis

- Hypothyroidism

- Hyperthyroidism

- Hypoparathyroidism; can affect calcium homeostasis, supplementation of which has completely resolved cases of depression in which hypoparathyroidism is the sole causative factor.

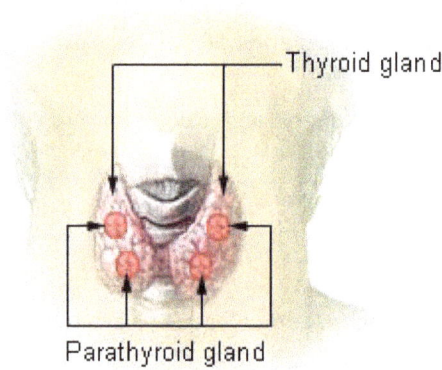

Thyroid gland

Parathyroid gland

Pituitary Tumors

Tumors of the pituitary gland are fairly common in the general population with estimates ranging as high as 25%. Most tumors are considered to be benign and are often an incidental finding discovered during autopsy or as of neuroimaging in which case they are dubbed "incidentalomas". Even in benign cases, pituitary tumors can affect cognitive, behavioral and emotional changes. Pituitary microadenomas are smaller than 10 mm in diameter and are generally considered benign, yet the presence of a microadenoma has been positively identified as a risk factor for suicide.

"patients with pituitary disease were diagnosed and treated for depression and showed little response to the treatment for depression".

Pancreas

- Hypoglycemia: an overproduction of insulin causes reduced blood levels of glucose. In one study of patients recovering from acute lung injury in intensive care, those patients who developed hypoglycemia while hospitalized showed an increased rate of depression.

Neurological

CNS Tumors

In addition to pituitary tumors, tumors in various locations in the central nervous system may cause depressive symptoms and be misdiagnosed as depression.

Post Concussion Syndrome

Post-concussion syndrome (PCS), is a set of symptoms that a person may experience for weeks, months, or occasionally years after a concussion with a prevalence rate of 38–80% in mild traumatic brain injuries, it may also occur in moderate and severe cases of traumatic brain injury. A diagnosis may be made when symptoms resulting from concussion, depending on criteria, last for more than three to six months after the injury, in which case it is termed persistent postconcussive syndrome (PPCS). In a study of the prevalence of post concussion syndrome symptoms in patients with depression utilizing the British Columbia Postconcussion Symptom Inventory: "Approximately 9 out of 10 patients with depression met liberal self-report criteria for a postconcussion syndrome and more than 5 out of 10 met conservative criteria for the diagnosis." These self reported rates were significantly higher than those obtained in a scheduled clinical interview. Normal controls have exhibited symptoms of PCS as well as those seeking psychological services. There is considerable debate over the diagnosis of PCS in part because of the medico-legal and thus monetary ramifications of receiving the diagnosis.

Pseudobulbar Affect

Characteristic	PBA	Depression
Duration	Seconds to minutes	Weeks to months
Voluntary control	None to minimal	Can be modulated by the situation
Affect	Unrelated to or independent of mood	Sad, worried, guilty, depressed; most often congruent with mood
Behavior	Does not change	Fatigued, apathetic, occasionally agitated
Perception	No misperceptions	Distorted and negative view of self, others, and future
Insight	Usually not impaired	May be impaired
Stimulus	Nonspecific, minimal or inappropriate to situation	Specific mood-related situations

Adapted from Cummings, 2007.

Diagnostic differences between PBA and depression

Pseudobulbar affect (PBA) is an affective disinhibition syndrome that is largely unrecognized in clinical settings and thus often untreated due to ignorance of the clinical manifestations of the disorder; it may be misdiagnosed as depression. It often occurs secondary to various neurodegenerative diseases such as amyotrophic lateral sclerosis, and also can result from head trauma. PBA is characterized by involuntary and inappropriate outbursts of laughter and/or crying. PBA has a high prevalence rate with estimates of 1.5–2 million cases in the United States alone.

Multiple Sclerosis

Multiple sclerosis is a chronic demyelinating disease in which the myelin sheaths of cells in the brain and spinal cord are irreparably damaged. Symptoms of depression are very common in patients at all stages of the disease and may be exacerbated by medical treatments, notably interferon beta-1a.

Neurotoxicity

Various compounds have been shown to have neurotoxic effects many of which have been implicated as having a causal relationship in the development of depression.

Cigarette Smoking

There has been research which suggests a correlation between cigarette smoking and depression. The results of one recent study suggest that smoking cigarettes may have a direct causal effect on the development of depression. There have been various studies done showing a positive link between smoking, suicidal ideation and suicide attempts.

In a study conducted among nurses, those smoking between 1-24 cigarettes per day had twice the suicide risk; 25 cigarettes or more, 4 times the suicide risk, than those who had never smoked. In a study of 300,000 male U.S. Army soldiers, a definitive link between suicide and smoking was observed with those smoking over a pack a day having twice the suicide rate of non-smokers.

Link Between Smoking Depression and Suicide

"Current daily smoking, but not past smoking, predicted the subsequent occurrence of suicidal thoughts or attempt."

"It would seem unwise, nevertheless, to rule out the possibility that smoking might be among the antecedent factors associated with the development of depression."

"Abstinence from cigarettes for prolonged periods may be associated with a decrease in depressive symptomatology."

"The stress induction model of smoking suggests, however, that smoking causes stress and concomitant negative affect."

Medication

Various medications have been suspected of having a causal relation in the development of depression; this has been classified as "organic mood syndrome". Some classes of medication such as those used to treat hypertension, have been recognized for decades as having a definitive relationship with the development of depression.

Monitoring of those taking medications which have shown a relationship with depression is often indicated, as well as the necessity of factoring in the use of such medications in the diagnostic process.

- Topical Tretinoin (Retin-A); derived from Vitamin A and used for various medical conditions such as in topical solutions used to treat acne vulgaris. Although applied externally to the skin, it may enter the bloodstream and cross the blood brain barrier where it may have neurotoxic effects.

- Interferons; proteins produced by the human body, three types have been identified *alpha, beta* and *gamma*. Synthetic versions are utilized in various medications used to treat different medical conditions such as the use of interferon-alpha in cancer treatment and hepatitis C treatment. All three classes of interferons may cause depression and suicidal ideation.

Chronic Exposure to Organophosphates

The neurophsychiatric effects of chronic organophosphate exposure include mood disorders, suicidal thinking and behaviour, cognitive impairment and chronic fatigue.

Neuropsychiatric

Bipolar disorder

- Bipolar disorder is frequently misdiagnosed as major depression, and is thus treated with antidepressants alone which is not only not efficacious it is often contraindicated as it may exacerbate hypomania, mania, or cycling between moods. There is ongoing debate about whether this should be classified as a separate disorder because individuals diagnosed with major depression often experience some hypomanic symptoms, indicating a continuum between the two.

Nutritional Deficiencies

Nutrition plays a key role in every facet of maintaining proper physical and psychological wellbeing. Insufficient or inadeqaute nutrition can have a profound effect on mental health. The emerging field of Nutritional Neuroscience explores the various connections between diet, neurological functioning and mental health.

- Vitamin B_6: pyridoxal phosphate (PLP), the active form of B_6, is a cofactor in the dopamine serotonin pathway, a deficiency in vitamin B_6 may cause depressive symptoms.

- Folate (vitamin B_9) – Vitamin B_{12} cobalamin: Low blood plasma and particularly red cell folate and diminished levels of vitamin B_{12} have been found in patients with depressive disorders. "We suggest that oral doses of both folic acid

(800 µg/(mcg) daily) and vitamin B12 (1 mg daily) should be tried to improve treatment outcome in depression."

- Long chain fatty acids: higher levels of omega-6 and lower levels of omega-3 fatty acids has been associated with depression and behavioral change.

- Vitamin D deficiency is associated with depression

Sleep Disorders

- Insomnia: While the inability to fall asleep is often a symptom of depression, it can also in some instances serve as the trigger for developing a depressive disorder. It can be transient, acute or chronic. It can be a primary disorder or a co-morbid one.

- Restless legs syndrome (RLS), also known as Wittmaack-Ekbom's syndrome, is characterized by an irresistible urge to move one's body to stop uncomfortable or odd sensations. It most commonly affects the legs, but can also affect the arms or torso, and even phantom limbs. Restless Leg syndrome has been associated with Major depressive disorder. "Adjusted odds ratio for diagnosis of major depressive disorder suggested a strong association between restless legs syndrome and major depressive disorder and/or panic disorder."

- Sleep apnea is a sleep disorder characterized by pauses in breathing during sleep. Each episode, called an apnea, lasts long enough for one or more breaths to be missed; such episodes occur repeatedly throughout the sleep cycle. Undiagnosed sleep apnea may cause or contribute to the severity of depression.

- Circadian rhythm sleep disorders, of which few clinicians are aware, often go untreated or are treated inappropriately, as when misdiagnosed as either primary insomnia or as a psychiatric condition.

Racing Thoughts

Racing thoughts refers to the rapid thought patterns that often occur in manic, hypomanic, or mixed episodes. While racing thoughts are most commonly described in people with bipolar disorder and sleep apnea, they are also common with anxiety disorders, OCD, and other psychiatric disorders such as attention deficit hyperactivity disorder. Racing thoughts are also associated with sleep deprivation, hyperthyroidism. and the use of amphetamines.

Description

Racing thoughts may be experienced as background or take over a person's consciousness. Thoughts, music, and voices might be zooming through one's mind as they jump tangentially from one to the next. There also might be a repetitive pattern of voice or of pressure without any associated "sound". It is a very overwhelming and irritating feeling, and can result in losing track of time. In some cases, it may also be frightening to the person experiencing it, as there is a loss of control. If one is experiencing these thoughts at night when going to sleep, they may suddenly awaken, startled and confused by the very random and sudden nature of the thoughts.

Racing thoughts differs in manifestation according to the individual's perspective. These manifestations can vary from unnoticed or minor distractions to debilitating stress, preventing the sufferer from maintaining a thought.

Generally, racing thoughts are described by an individual who has had an episode where the mind uncontrollably brings up random thoughts and memories and switches between them very quickly. Sometimes they are related, as one thought leads to another; other times they seem completely random. A person suffering from an episode of racing thoughts has no control over his or her train of thought, and it stops them from focusing on one topic or prevents sleeping.

Associated Conditions

The causes of racing thoughts are most often associated with anxiety disorders, but many influences can cause these rapid, racing thoughts. There are also many associated conditions, in addition to anxiety disorders, which can be classified as having secondary relationships with causing racing thoughts. The conditions most commonly linked to racing thoughts are bipolar disorder, anxiety disorder, attention deficit hyperactivity disorder, sleep deprivation, amphetamine dependence, and hyperthyroidism.

Anxiety Disorder

Racing thoughts associated with anxiety disorder can be caused by many different conditions, such as Obsessive Compulsive Disorder OCD, panic disorder, schizophrenia, general anxiety disorder (GAD), or posttraumatic stress disorder.

In people with OCD, racing thoughts can be brought on by stressors, or triggers, causing disturbing thoughts in the individual. These disturbing thoughts, then, result in compulsions characterizing OCD in order to lower the stress and gain some sort of control over these stressful, racing thoughts.

Panic disorder is an anxiety disorder characterized by repeated panic attacks of fear or nervousness, lasting several minutes. During these panic attacks, the response is out of proportion to the situation. The racing thoughts may feel catastrophic and intense, but they are a symptom of the panic attack and must be controlled in order to soothe the panic and minimize the panic attack.

Schizophrenia is defined by many different behavioral, physical and cognitive symptoms. Many of the cognitive symptoms involve racing and obsessive thoughts. Racing thoughts ruminate over and over, most likely about past failures or disappointments. Thoughts that seem to not have a clear association with each other and do not logically connect are associated with schizophrenia. Racing thoughts, in general, are a symptom of this mental disorder. There are also many other cognitive symptoms that involve obsessive and rapid ideas which lead to illogical and nonsensical racing thoughts.

General anxiety disorder is a neurological anxiety disorder that involves uncontrollable and excessive worrying about irrational topics or problems. These stressful thoughts must be present for at least six months in order to be diagnosed as GAD. Along with other symptoms, racing thoughts is one of the most common ones. With GAD, there is an inability to relax or let thoughts or worries go, persistent worrying and obsessions about small concerns that are out of proportion to the result, and even worrying about their excessive worrying.

Bipolar Disorder

Racing thoughts can be brought on by bipolar disorder, defined by mood instability that ranges from extreme emotional highs, mania, to severe depression. During the manic phase of bipolar disorder is when racing thoughts usually occur. Disjointed, constantly changing thoughts with no underlying theme can be a sign of the manic phase of bipolar disorder. Manic thoughts can prevent performance of daily routines due to the rapid, manic thoughts. Racing thoughts in people with bipolar disorder are generally accompanied with other symptoms associated with this disorder.

Amphetamines

Amphetamines are used as a stimulant to trigger the central nervous system, increasing heart rate and blood pressure while decreasing appetite. Since amphetamines are a stimulant, use of these drugs result in a state that resembles the manic phase of bipolar disorder and also produces similar symptoms, as stated above.

Attention Deficit Hyperactivity Disorder

Racing thoughts associated with ADHD is most common in adults. With ADHD, racing thoughts can occur and tend to cause insomnia. Racing thoughts in people with ADHD tend to be rapid, unstable thoughts which do not follow any sort of pattern, similar to racing thoughts in people with bipolar disorder. Medications used to treat ADHD, such as Adderall or Ritalin, can be prescribed to patients to calm these and other symptoms caused by ADHD.

Lack of Sleep

Racing thoughts, also referred to as "racing mind", may prevent a person from falling asleep. Chronic sleep apnea and prolonged disturbed sleep patterns may also induce racing thoughts. Treatment for sleep apnea and obstructive airway disorder can improve airflow and improve sleep resulting in improved brain and REM function and reduced racing thought patterns.

Hyperthyroidism

Hyperthyroidism is a condition in which the thyroid gland produces too much thyroid hormone, thyroxin. This overabundance of thyroxin causes irregular and rapid heartbeat, irritability, weight loss, nervousness, anxiety and racing thoughts. The anxiety and inability to focus is very common in hyperthyroidism and leads to racing thoughts, as well as panic attacks and difficulty concentrating.

Frequency

Anxiety disorder, the most common mental illness in the United States, affects 40 million people, ages 18 and older; this accounts for 18% of the U.S. population. Most people suffering from anxiety disorder report some form of racing thoughts symptom

The prevalence of OCD in every culture studied is at least 2% of the population, and the majority of those have obsessions, or racing thoughts. With these reportings, estimates of more than 2 million people in the United States (as of 2000) suffer from racing thoughts.

Treatment

There are various treatments available to calm racing thoughts, some of which involve medication. One type of treatment involves writing out the thoughts onto paper. Some treatments suggest using activities, such as painting, cooking, and other hobbies, to keep the mind busy and distract from the racing thoughts. Exercise may be used to tire the person, thereby calming their mind. When racing thoughts are anxiety induced during panic or anxiety attacks, it is recommended that the person wait it out. Using breathing and meditation techniques to calm the breath and mind simultaneously is another tool for handling racing thoughts induced by anxiety attacks. Mindfulness meditation has also shown to help with racing thoughts by allowing practitioners to face their thoughts head-on, without reacting.

While all of these techniques can be useful to cope with racing thoughts, it may prove necessary to seek medical attention and counsel. Since racing thoughts are associated with many other underlying mental illnesses, such as bipolar disorder, anxiety disorder, and ADHD, medications used commonly to treat these disorders will help calm racing thoughts in patients.

Treatment for the underlying causes of racing thoughts is helpful and useful in order to calm the racing thoughts more permanently. For example, in people with ADHD, medications used to promote focus and calm distracting thoughts, will help them with their ADHD. Also, people with insomnia who have resulting racing thoughts will find Sleep Apnea treatment & Nasal surgery helpful to eliminate their racing thoughts. It is important to look at the underlying defect that may be causing your racing thoughts in order to prevent them long-term.

References

- Leo P. W. Chiu (1989). "Differential diagnosis and management of hallucinations" (PDF). Journal of the Hong Kong Medical Association. t 41 (3): 292–7

- Panayiotopoulos CP (2007). A clinical guide to epileptic syndromes and their treatment (2nd ed.). London: Springer. ISBN 978-1846286438. based on the ILAE classification and practice parameter guidelines

- Joseph M. Tonkonogy, Iosif Moiseevich Tonkonogiĭ, Antonio E. Puente (2009). Localization of Clinical Syndromes in Neuropsychology and Neuroscience. Springer. p. 200. ISBN 0826119670. Retrieved July 11, 2012

- Knoll, James L., Resnick, Phillip J. (2008). "Insanity Defense Evaluations: Toward a Model for Evidence-Based Practice". Brief Treatment and Crisis Intervention. 8 (1): 92–110. doi:10.1093/brief-treatment/mhm024

- Barker P (1997). Assessment in psychiatric and mental health nursing: in search of the whole person. Cheltenham, UK: Stanley Thornes Publishers. p. 245. ISBN 978-0748731749

- Leone, Caterina; Biasiotta, Antonella. "Pathophysiological Mechanisms of Neuropathic Pain". Medscape. Retrieved 7 August 2014

- Leopold, D. A. (2002), "Distortion of Olfactory Perception: Diagnosis and Treatment", Chemical Senses, 27 (7): 611–615, PMID 12200340, doi:10.1093/chemse/27.7.611

- Chakrabarty A, Reddy MS (2011). "Visual hallucinations in mania". Indian Journal of Psychological Medicine. 33 (1): 71–73. PMC 3195159. PMID 22021957. doi:10.4103/0253-7176.85399

- Horowitz MJ (1975). "Hallucinations: An Information Processing Approach". In West LJ, Siegel RK. Hallucinations; behavior, experience, and theory. New York: Wiley. ISBN 0-471-79096-6

- Author, UTHSCSA Dental School CATs. "UTCAT2395, Found CAT view, CRITICALLY APPRAISED TOPICs". cats.uthscsa.edu. Retrieved 2016-03-08

- Sim L., Zeman J. (2006). "The contribution of emotion regulation to body dissatisfaction and disordered eating in early adolescent girls". Journal of Youth and Adolescence. 2: 207–216

- Hockenbury, Don and Sandra (2011). Discovering Psychology Fifth Edition. New York, NY: Worth Publishers. p. 549. ISBN 978-1-4292-1650-0

- Wollenberg, Anne (July 28, 2008). "Time to wake up to sleep disorders". Guardian News and Media Limited. Retrieved 2008-08-03

- Friedrich F, Geusau A, Greisenegger S, Ossege M, Aigner M (2009). "Manifest psychosis in neurosyphilis". General Hospital Psychiatry. 31 (4): 379–81. PMID 19555800. doi:10.1016/j.genhosppsych.2008.09.010

- Hauri, PJ; Silber, MH; Boeve, BF (2007). "The treatment of parasomnias with hypnosis: A

5-year follow-up study". Journal of Clinical Sleep Medicine. 3 (4): 369–73. PMC 1978312. PMID 17694725

- "Hyperthyroidism (overactive thyroid)". MayoClinic. Mayo Foundation for Medical Education and Research. 2014. Retrieved November 11, 2014

- Catassi C (2015). "Gluten Sensitivity.". Ann Nutr Metab (Review). 67 Suppl 2: 16–26. PMID 26605537. doi:10.1159/000440990

- Ohayon MM (Dec 2000). "Prevalence of hallucinations and their pathological associations in the general population". Psychiatry Res. 97 (2–3): 153–64. PMID 11166087. doi:10.1016/S0165-1781(00)00227-4

- Lee TM, Chong SA, Chan YH, Sathyadevan G (2004). "Command hallucinations among Asian patients with schizophrenia". Canadian Journal of Psychiatry. 49 (12): 838–42. PMID 15679207

Anxiety Disorder: An Integrated Study

Anxiety disorders are a group of mental disorders whose symptoms include anxiety and fear. Individuals often exhibit a variety of anxiety disorders and phobias at the same time. Mood disorders are best understood in confluence with the major topics listed in the following chapter.

Anxiety Disorder

Anxiety disorders are a group of mental disorders characterized by feelings of anxiety and fear. Anxiety is a worry about future events and fear is a reaction to current events. These feelings may cause physical symptoms, such as a fast heart rate and shakiness. There are a number of anxiety disorders: including generalized anxiety disorder, specific phobia, social anxiety disorder, separation anxiety disorder, agoraphobia, panic disorder, and selective mutism. The disorder differs by what results in the symptoms. People often have more than one anxiety disorder.

The cause of anxiety disorders is a combination of genetic and environmental factors. Risk factors include a history of child abuse, family history of mental disorders, and poverty. Anxiety disorders often occur with other mental disorders, particularly major depressive disorder, personality disorder, and substance use disorder. To be diagnosed symptoms typically need to be present for at least six months, be more than would be expected for the situation, and decrease functioning. Other problems that may result in similar symptoms including hyperthyroidism; heart disease; caffeine, alcohol, or cannabis use; and withdrawal from certain drugs, among others.

Without treatment, anxiety disorders tend to remain. Treatment may include lifestyle changes, counselling, and medications. Counselling is typically with a type of cognitive behavioural therapy. Medications, such as antidepressants or beta blockers, may improve symptoms.

About 12% of people are affected by an anxiety disorder in a given year and between 5-30% are affected at some point in their life. They occur about twice as often in females as males, and generally begin before the age of 25. The most common are specific phobia which affects nearly 12% and social anxiety disorder which affects 10% at some point in their life. They affect those between the ages of 15 and 35 the most and become less common after the age of 55. Rates appear to be higher in the United States and Europe.

Classification

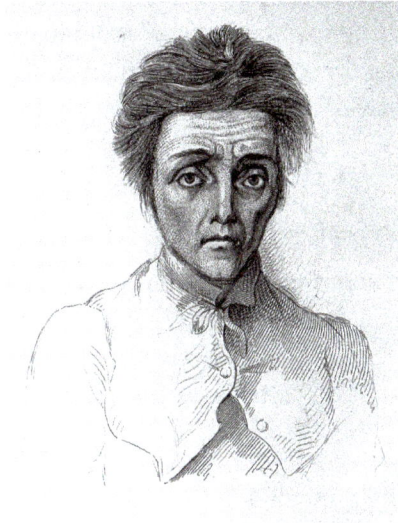

Facial expression of someone with chronic anxiety

Generalized Anxiety Disorder

Generalized anxiety disorder (GAD) is a common disorder, characterized by long-lasting anxiety that is not focused on any one object or situation. Those suffering from generalized anxiety disorder experience non-specific persistent fear and worry, and become overly concerned with everyday matters. Generalized anxiety disorder is "characterized by chronic excessive worry accompanied by three or more of the following symptoms: restlessness, fatigue, concentration problems, irritability, muscle tension, and sleep disturbance". Generalized anxiety disorder is the most common anxiety disorder to affect older adults. Anxiety can be a symptom of a medical or substance abuse problem, and medical professionals must be aware of this. A diagnosis of GAD is made when a person has been excessively worried about an everyday problem for six months or more. A person may find that they have problems making daily decisions and remembering commitments as a result of lack of concentration/preoccupation with worry. Appearance looks strained, with increased sweating from the hands, feet, and axillae, and they may be tearful, which can suggest depression. Before a diagnosis of anxiety disorder is made, physicians must rule out drug-induced anxiety and other medical causes.

In children GAD may be associated with headaches, restlessness, abdominal pain, and heart palpitations. Typically it begins around 8 to 9 years of age.

Specific Phobias

The single largest category of anxiety disorders is that of specific phobias which includes all cases in which fear and anxiety are triggered by a specific stimulus or situation. Between 5% and 12% of the population worldwide suffer from specific phobias. Sufferers typically anticipate terrifying consequences from encountering the object of their fear, which can be anything from an animal to a location to a bodily fluid to a particular situation. Sufferers understand that their fear is not proportional to the actual potential danger but still are overwhelmed by it.

Panic Disorder

With panic disorder, a person has brief attacks of intense terror and apprehension, often marked by trembling, shaking, confusion, dizziness, nausea, and/or difficulty breathing. These panic attacks, defined by the APA as fear or discomfort that abruptly arises and peaks in less than ten minutes, can last for several hours. Attacks can be triggered by stress, fear, or even exercise; the specific cause is not always apparent.

In addition to recurrent unexpected panic attacks, a diagnosis of panic disorder requires that said attacks have chronic consequences: either worry over the attacks' potential implications, persistent fear of future attacks, or significant changes in behavior related to the attacks. As such, those suffering from panic disorder experience symptoms even outside specific panic episodes. Often, normal changes in heartbeat are noticed by a panic sufferer, leading them to think something is wrong with their heart or they are about to have another panic attack. In some cases, a heightened awareness (hypervigilance) of body functioning occurs during panic attacks, wherein any perceived physiological change is interpreted as a possible life-threatening illness (i.e., extreme hypochondriasis).

Agoraphobia

Agoraphobia is the specific anxiety about being in a place or situation where escape is difficult or embarrassing or where help may be unavailable. Agoraphobia is strongly linked with panic disorder and is often precipitated by the fear of having a panic attack. A common manifestation involves needing to be in constant view of a door or other escape route. In addition to the fears themselves, the term agoraphobia is often used to refer to avoidance behaviors that sufferers often develop. For example, following a panic attack while driving, someone suffering from agoraphobia may develop anxiety over driving and will therefore avoid driving. These avoidance behaviors can often have serious consequences and often reinforce the fear they are caused by.

Social Anxiety Disorder

Social anxiety disorder (SAD; also known as social phobia) describes an intense fear and avoidance of negative public scrutiny, public embarrassment, humiliation, or social interaction. This fear can be specific to particular social situations (such as public speaking) or, more typically, is experienced in most (or all) social interactions. Social anxiety often manifests specific physical symptoms, including blushing, sweating, and difficulty speaking. As with all phobic disorders, those suffering from social anxiety often will attempt to avoid the source of their anxiety; in the case of social anxiety this is particularly problematic, and in severe cases can lead to complete social isolation.

Social physique anxiety (SPA) is a subtype of social anxiety. It is concern over the evaluation of one's body by others. SPA is common among adolescents, especially females.

Post-traumatic Stress Disorder

Post-traumatic stress disorder (PTSD) is an anxiety disorder that results from a traumatic experience. Post-traumatic stress can result from an extreme situation, such as combat, natural disaster, rape, hostage situations, child abuse, bullying, or even a serious accident. It can also result from long-term (chronic) exposure to a severe stressor-- for example, soldiers who endure individual battles but cannot cope with continuous combat. Common symptoms include hypervigilance, flashbacks, avoidant behaviors, anxiety, anger and depression. There are a number of treatments that form the basis of the care plan for those suffering with PTSD. Such treatments include cognitive behavioral therapy (CBT), psychotherapy and support from family and friends.

Posttraumatic stress disorder (PTSD) research began with Vietnam veterans, as well as natural and non natural disaster victims. Studies have found the degree of exposure to a disaster has been found to be the best predictor of PTSD.

Separation Anxiety Disorder

Separation anxiety disorder (SepAD) is the feeling of excessive and inappropriate levels of anxiety over being separated from a person or place. Separation anxiety is a normal part of development in babies or children, and it is only when this feeling is excessive or inappropriate that it can be considered a disorder. Separation anxiety disorder affects roughly 7% of adults and 4% of children, but the childhood cases tend to be more severe; in some instances, even a brief separation can produce panic. Treating a child earlier may prevent problems. This may include training the parents and family on how to deal with it. Often, the parents will reinforce the anxiety because they do not know how to properly work through it with the child. In addition to parent training and family therapy, medication, such as SSRIs, can be used to treat separation anxiety.

Situational Anxiety

Situational anxiety is caused by new situations or changing events. It can also be caused by various events that make that particular individual uncomfortable. Its occurrence is very common. Often, an individual will experience panic attacks or extreme anxiety in specific situations. A situation that causes one individual to experience anxiety may not affect another individual at all. For example, some people become uneasy in crowds or tight spaces, so standing in a tightly packed line, say at the bank or a store register, may cause them to experience extreme anxiety, possibly a panic attack. Others, however, may experience anxiety when major changes in life occur, such as entering college, getting married, having children, etc.

Obsessive–compulsive Disorder

Obsessive–compulsive disorder (OCD) is not classified as an anxiety disorder by the DSM-5 but is by the ICD-10. It was previously classified as an anxiety disorder in the DSM-IV. It is a condition where the person has obsessions (distressing, persistent, and intrusive thoughts or images) and/or compulsions (urges to repeatedly perform specific acts or rituals), that are not caused by drugs or physical order, and which cause distress or social dysfunction. The compulsive rituals are personal rules followed to relieve the anxiety. OCD affects roughly 1-2% of adults (somewhat more women than men), and under 3% of children and adolescents.

A person with OCD knows that the symptoms are unreasonable and struggles against both the thoughts and the behavior. Their symptoms could be related to external events they fear (such as their home burning down because they forget to turn off the stove) or worry that they will behave inappropriately.

It is not certain why some people have OCD, but behavioral, cognitive, genetic, and neurobiological factors may be involved. Risk factors include family history, being single (although that may result from the disorder), and higher socioeconomic class or not being in paid employment. OCD is chronic; about 20% of people will overcome it, and symptoms will at least reduce over time for most people (a further 50%).

Selective Mutism

Selective mutism (SM) is a disorder in which a person who is normally capable of speech does not speak in specific situations or to specific people. Selective mutism usually co-exists with shyness or social anxiety. People with selective mutism stay silent even when the consequences of their silence include shame, social ostracism or even punishment. Selective mutism affects about 0.8% of people at some point in their life.

Causes

Drugs

Anxiety and depression can be caused by alcohol abuse, which in most cases improves with prolonged abstinence. Even moderate, sustained alcohol use may increase anxiety levels in some individuals. Caffeine, alcohol and benzodiazepine dependence can worsen or cause anxiety and panic attacks. Anxiety commonly occurs during the acute withdrawal phase of alcohol and can persist for up to 2 years as part of a post-acute withdrawal syndrome, in about a quarter of people recovering from alcoholism. In one study in 1988–1990, illness in approximately half of patients attending mental health services at one British hospital psychiatric clinic, for conditions including anxiety disorders such as panic disorder or social phobia, was determined to be the result of alcohol or benzodiazepine dependence. In these patients, an initial increase in anxiety occurred during the withdrawal period followed by a cessation of their anxiety symptoms.

There is evidence that chronic exposure to organic solvents in the work environment can be associated with anxiety disorders. Painting, varnishing and carpet-laying are some of the jobs in which significant exposure to organic solvents may occur.

Taking caffeine may cause or worsen anxiety disorders, including panic disorder. Those with anxiety disorders can have high caffeine sensitivity. Caffeine-induced anxiety disorder is a subclass of the DSM-5 diagnosis of substance/medication-induced anxiety disorder. Substance/medication-induced anxiety disorder falls under the category of anxiety disorders, and not the category of substance-related and addictive disorders, even though the symptoms are due to the effects of a substance.

Cannabis use is associated with anxiety disorders. However, the precise relationship between cannabis use and anxiety still needs to be established.

Medical Conditions

Occasionally, an anxiety disorder may be a side-effect of an underlying endocrine disease that causes nervous system hyperactivity, such as pheochromocytoma or hyperthyroidism.

Stress

Anxiety disorders can arise in response to life stresses such as financial worries or chronic physical illness. Anxiety among adolescents and young adults is common due to the stresses of social interaction, evaluation, and body image. Anxiety is also common among older people who have dementia. On the other hand, anxiety disorder is sometimes misdiagnosed among older adults when doctors misinterpret symptoms of a physical ailment (for instance, racing heartbeat due to cardiac arrhythmia) as signs of anxiety.

Genetics

GAD runs in families and is six times more common in the children of someone with the condition.

While anxiety arose as an adaptation, in modern times it is almost always thought of negatively in the context of anxiety disorders. People with these disorders have highly sensitive systems; hence, their systems tend to overreact to seemingly harmless stimuli. Sometimes anxiety disorders occur in those who have had traumatic youths, demonstrating an increased prevalence of anxiety when it appears a child will have a difficult future. In these cases, the disorder arises as a way to predict that the individual's environment will continue to pose threats.

Persistence of Anxiety

At a low level, anxiety is not a bad thing. In fact, the hormonal response to anxiety has evolved as a benefit, as it helps humans react to dangers. Researchers in evolutionary medicine believe this adaptation allows humans to realize there is a potential threat and to act accordingly in order to ensure greatest possibility of protection. It has actually been shown that those with low levels of anxiety have a greater risk of death than those with average levels. This is because the absence of fear can lead to injury or death. Additionally, patients with both anxiety and depression were found to have lower morbidity than those with depression alone. The functional significance of the symptoms associated with anxiety includes: greater alertness, quicker preparation for action, and reduced probability of missing threats. In the wild, vulnerable individuals, for example those who are hurt or pregnant, have a lower threshold for anxiety response, making them more alert. This demonstrates a lengthy evolutionary history of the anxiety response.

Evolutionary Mismatch

It has been theorized that high rates of anxiety are a reaction to how the social environment has changed from the Paleolithic era. For example, in the Stone Age there was greater skin-to-skin contact and more handling of babies by their mothers, both of which are strategies that reduce anxiety. Additionally, there is greater interaction with strangers in present times as opposed to interactions solely between close-knit tribes. Researchers posit that the lack of constant social interaction, especially in the formative years, is a driving cause of high rates of anxiety.

Many current cases are likely to have resulted from an evolutionary mismatch, which has been specifically termed a "psychopathogical mismatch". In evolutionary terms, a mismatch occurs when an individual possesses traits that were adapted for an environment that differs from the individual's current environment. For example, even though an anxiety reaction may have been evolved to help with life-threatening situations, for highly sensitized individuals in Westernized cultures simply hearing bad news can elicit a strong reaction.

An evolutionary perspective may provide insight into alternatives to current clinical treatment methods for anxiety disorders. Simply knowing some anxiety is beneficial may alleviate some of the panic associated with mild conditions. Some researchers believe that, in theory, anxiety can be mediated by reducing a patient's feeling of vulnerability and then changing their appraisal of the situation.

Mechanisms

Biological

Low levels of GABA, a neurotransmitter that reduces activity in the central nervous system, contribute to anxiety. A number of anxiolytics achieve their effect by modulating the GABA receptors.

Selective serotonin reuptake inhibitors, the drugs most commonly used to treat depression, are frequently considered as a first line treatment for anxiety disorders.

Amygdala

The amygdala is central to the processing of fear and anxiety, and its function may be disrupted in anxiety disorders. Sensory information enters the amygdala through the nuclei of the basolateral complex (consisting of lateral, basal, and accessory basal nuclei). The basolateral complex processes sensory-related fear memories and communicates their threat importance to memory and sensory processing elsewhere in the brain, such as the medial prefrontal cortex and sensory cortices.

Another important area is the adjacent central nucleus of the amygdala, which controls species-specific fear responses, via connections to the brainstem, hypothalamus, and cerebellum areas. In those with general anxiety disorder, these connections functionally seem to be less distinct, with greater gray matter in the central nucleus. Another difference is that the amygdala areas have decreased connectivity with the insula and cingulate areas that control general stimulus salience, while having greater connectivity with the parietal cortex and prefrontal cortex circuits that underlie executive functions.

The latter suggests a compensation strategy for dysfunctional amygdala processing of anxiety. Researchers have noted "Amygdalofrontoparietal coupling in generalized anxiety disorder patients may ... reflect the habitual engagement of a cognitive control system to regulate excessive anxiety." This is consistent with cognitive theories that suggest the use in this disorder of attempts to reduce the involvement of emotions with compensatory cognitive strategies.

Clinical and animal studies suggest a correlation between anxiety disorders and difficulty in maintaining balance. A possible mechanism is malfunction in the parabrachial area, a brain structure that, among other functions, coordinates signals from the amygdala with input concerning balance.

Anxiety processing in the basolateral amygdala has been implicated with dendritic arborization of the amygdaloid neurons. SK2 potassium channels mediate inhibitory influence on action potentials and reduce arborization. By overexpressing SK2 in the basolateral amygdala, anxiety in experimental animals can be reduced together with general levels of stress-induced corticosterone secretion.

Prevention

Focus is increasing on prevention of anxiety disorders. There is tentative evidence to support the use of cognitive behavior therapy and mindfulness therapy. As of 2013, there are no effective measures to prevent GAD in adults.

Diagnosis

Anxiety disorders are often severe chronic conditions, which can be present from an early age or begin suddenly after a triggering event. They are prone to flare up at times of high stress and are frequently accompanied by physiological symptoms such as headache, sweating, muscle spasms, tachycardia, palpitations, and hypertension, which in some cases lead to fatigue.

In casual discourse the words "anxiety" and "fear" are often used interchangeably; in clinical usage, they have distinct meanings: "anxiety" is defined as an unpleasant emotional state for which the cause is either not readily identified or perceived to be uncontrollable or unavoidable, whereas "fear" is an emotional and physiological response to a recognized external threat. The term "anxiety disorder" includes fears (phobias) as well as anxieties.

The diagnosis of anxiety disorders is difficult because there are no objective biomarkers, it is based on symptoms, which typically need to be present at least six months, be more than would be expected for the situation, and decrease functioning. Several generic anxiety questionnaires can be used to detect anxiety symptoms, such as the State-Trait Anxiety Inventory (STAI), the Generalized Anxiety Disorder 7 (GAD-7), the Beck Anxiety Inventory (BAI), the Zung Self-Rating Anxiety Scale, and the Taylor Manifest Anxiety Scale. Other questionnaires combine anxiety and depression measurement, such as the Hamilton Anxiety Rating Scale, the Hospital Anxiety and Depression Scale (HADS), the Patient Health Questionnaire (PHQ), and the Patient-Reported Outcomes Measurement Information System (PROMIS). Examples of specific anxiety questionnaires include the Liebowitz Social Anxiety Scale (LSAS), the Social Interaction Anxiety Scale (SIAS), the Social Phobia Inventory (SPIN), the Social Phobia Scale (SPS), and the Social Anxiety Questionnaire (SAQ-A30).

Anxiety disorders often occur along with other mental disorders, in particular depression, which may occur in as many as 60% of people with anxiety disorders. The fact that there is considerable overlap between symptoms of anxiety and depression, and that the same environmental triggers can provoke symptoms in either condition, may help to explain this high rate of comorbidity.

Studies have also indicated that anxiety disorders are more likely among those with family history of anxiety disorders, especially certain types.

Sexual dysfunction often accompanies anxiety disorders, although it is difficult to determine whether anxiety causes the sexual dysfunction or whether they arise from a common cause. The most common manifestations in individuals with anxiety disorder are avoidance of intercourse, premature ejaculation or erectile dysfunction among men and pain during intercourse among women. Sexual dysfunction is particularly common among people affected by panic disorder (who may fear that a panic attack will occur during sexual arousal) and posttraumatic stress disorder.

Differential Diagnosis

The diagnosis of an anxiety disorder requires first ruling out an underlying medical cause. Diseases that may present similar to an anxiety disorder, including certain endocrine diseases (hypo- and hyperthyroidism, hyperprolactinemia), metabolic disorders (diabetes), deficiency states (low levels of vitamin D, B2, B12, folic acid), gastrointestinal diseases (celiac disease, non-celiac gluten sensitivity, inflammatory bowel disease), heart diseases, blood diseases (anemia), and brain degenerative diseases (Parkinson's disease, dementia, multiple sclerosis, Huntington's disease).

Also, several drugs can cause or worsen anxiety, whether in intoxication, withdrawal, or from chronic use. These include alcohol, tobacco, cannabis, sedatives (including prescription benzodiazepines), opioids (including prescription pain killers and illicit drugs like heroin), stimulants (such as caffeine, cocaine and amphetamines), hallucinogens, and inhalants.

Treatment

Treatment options include lifestyle changes, therapy, and medications. There is no good evidence as to whether therapy or medication is more effective; the choice of which is up to the person with the anxiety disorder and most choose therapy first. The other may be offered in addition to the first choice or if the first choice fails to relieve symptoms.

Lifestyle Changes

Lifestyle changes include exercise, for which there is moderate evidence for some improvement, regularizing sleep patterns, reducing caffeine intake, and stopping smoking. Stopping smoking has benefits in anxiety as large as or larger than those of medications.

Therapy

Cognitive behavioral therapy (CBT) is effective for anxiety disorders and is a first line treatment. CBT appears to be equally effective when carried out via the internet. While evidence for mental health apps is promising it is preliminary.

Self-help books can contribute to the treatment of people with anxiety disorders.

Mindfulness based programs also appear to be effective for managing anxiety disorders. It is unclear if meditation has an effect on anxiety and transcendental meditation appears to be no different than other types of meditation.

Medications

Medications include SSRIs or SNRIs are first line choices for generalized anxiety disorder; there is no good evidence for any member of the class being better than another, so cost often drives drug choice. Buspirone, quetiapine and pregabalin are second line treatments for people who do not respond to SSRIs or SNRIs; there is also evidence that benzodiazepines including diazepam and clonazepam are effective but have fallen out of favor due to the risk of dependence and abuse.

Medications need to be used with care among older adults, who are more likely to have side effects because of coexisting physical disorders. Adherence problems are more likely among older people, who may have difficulty understanding, seeing, or remembering instructions.

In general medications are not seen as helpful in specific phobia but a benzodiazepine is sometimes used to help resolve acute episodes; as 2007 data were sparse for efficacy of any drug.

Alternative Medicine

Many other remedies have been used for anxiety disorder. These include kava, where the potential for benefit seems greater than that for harm with short-term use in those with mild to moderate anxiety. The American Academy of Family Physicians (AAFP) recommends use of kava for those with mild to moderate anxiety disorders who are not using alcohol or taking other medicines metabolized by the liver, and who wish to use "natural" remedies. Side effects of kava in the clinical trials were rare and mild.

Inositol has been found to have modest effects in people with panic disorder or obsessive-compulsive disorder. There is insufficient evidence to support the use of St. John's wort, valerian or passionflower.

Aromatherapy has shown some tentative benefits for anxiety reduction in people with cancer when done with massages, although it not clear whether it could just enhance the effect of massage itself.

Children

Several methods of treatment have been found to be effective in treating childhood anxiety disorders. Therapy is strongly preferred to medication.

Cognitive behavioral therapy (CBT), a well-established treatment for anxiety related disorders in children and adolescents, is a good first therapy approach. Studies have also gathered substantial evidence for treatments that are not CBT based as being effective forms of treament, expanding treatment options for those who do not respond to CBT. Like adults, children may undergo psychotherapy, cognitive-behavioral therapy, or counseling. Family therapy is a form of treatment in which the child meets with a therapist together with the primary guardians and siblings. Each family member may attend individual therapy, but family therapy is typically a form of group therapy. Art and play therapy are also used. Art therapy is most commonly used when the child will not or cannot verbally communicate, due to trauma or a disability in which they are nonverbal. Participating in art activities allows the child to express what they otherwise may not be able to communicate to others. In play therapy, the child is allowed to play however they please as a therapist observes them. The therapist may intercede from time to time with a question, comment, or suggestion. This is often most effective when the family of the child plays a role in the treatment.

In children and adolescents, a medication option is warranted, antidepressants such as SSRIs, SNRIs as well as tricyclic antidepressants can be effective.

Prognosis

The prognosis varies on the severity of each case and utilization of treatment for each individual.

If these children are left untreated, they face risks such as poor results at school, avoidance of important social activities, and substance abuse. Children who have an anxiety disorder are likely to have other disorders such as depression, eating disorders, attention deficit disorders both hyperactive and inattentive.

Epidemiology

Globally as of 2010 approximately 273 million (4.5% of the population) had an anxiety disorder. It is more common in females (5.2%) than males (2.8%).

In Europe, Africa and Asia, lifetime rates of anxiety disorders are between 9 and 16%, and yearly rates are between 4 and 7%. In the United States, the lifetime prevalence of anxiety disorders is about 29% and between 11 and 18% of adults have the condition in a given year. This difference is affected by the range of ways in which different cultures interpret anxiety symptoms and what they consider to be normative behavior. In general, anxiety disorders represent the most prevalent psychiatric condition in the United States, outside of substance use disorder.

Children

Like adults, children can experience anxiety disorders; between 10 and 20 percent of all children will develop a full-fledged anxiety disorder prior to the age of 18, making anxiety the most common mental health issue in young people. Anxiety disorders in children are often more challenging to identify than their adult counterparts owing to the difficulty many parents face in discerning them from normal childhood fears. Likewise, anxiety in children is sometimes misdiagnosed as an attention deficit disorder or, due to the tendency of children to interpret their emotions physically (as stomach aches, head aches, etc.), anxiety disorders may initially be confused with physical ailments.

Anxiety in children has a variety of causes; sometimes anxiety is rooted in biology, and may be a product of another existing condition, such as autism or Asperger's disorder. Gifted children are also often more prone to excessive anxiety than non-gifted children. Other cases of anxiety arise from the child having experienced a traumatic event of some kind, and in some cases, the cause of the child's anxiety cannot be pinpointed.

Anxiety in children tends to manifest along age-appropriate themes, such as fear of going to school (not related to bullying) or not performing well enough at school, fear of social rejection, fear of something happening to loved ones, etc. What separates disordered anxiety from normal childhood anxiety is the duration and intensity of the fears involved.

A small child will usually experience separation anxiety, for example, but he or she will generally grow out of it by about the age of 6, whereas in an anxious child it may linger for years longer, hindering the child's development. Similarly, most children will fear the dark or losing their parents at some point, but this fear will dissipate over time without interfering a great deal in that child's normal day-to-day activities. In a child with an anxiety disorder, fearing the dark or loss of loved ones may grow into a lasting obsession which the child tries to deal with in compulsive ways which erode his or her quality of life. The presence of co- occurring depressive symptoms in anxiety disorders may mark the transition to a more severe and detrimental and impairing disorder in preschool and early school age.

Children, similar to adults, may suffer from a range of different anxiety disorders, including:

Generalized anxiety disorder: The child experiences persistent anxiety regarding a wide variety of situations, and this anxiety may adapt to fit each new situation that arises or be based largely on imagined situations which have yet to occur. Reassurance often has little effect.

Separation anxiety disorder: A child who is older than 6 or 7 who has an extremely difficult time being away from his or her parents may be experiencing Separation Anxiety Disorder. Children with this disorder often fear that they will lose their loved ones during times of absence. As such, they frequently refuse to attend school.

Social anxiety disorder should not be confused with shyness or introversion; shyness is frequently normal, especially in very young children. Children with social anxiety disorder often wish to engage in social activity (unlike introverts) but find themselves held back by obsessive fears of being disliked. They often convince themselves they have made a poor impression on others, regardless of evidence to the contrary. Over time, they may develop a phobia of social situations. This disorder affects older children and preteens more often than younger children. Social phobia in children may also be caused by some traumatic event, such as not knowing an answer when called on in class.

While uncommon in children, OCD can occur. Rates are between two and four percent. Like adults, children rely on "magical thinking" in order to allay their anxiety, i.e., he or she must perform certain rituals (often based in counting, organizing, cleaning, etc.) in order to "prevent" the calamity he or she feels is imminent. Unlike normal children, who can leave their magical thinking-based activities behind when called upon to do so, children with OCD are literally unable to cease engaging in these activities, regardless of the consequences.

Panic disorder is more common in older children, though younger children sometimes also suffer from it. Panic disorder is frequently mistaken for a physical illness by children suffering from it, likely due to its strongly physical symptoms (a racing heartbeat, sweating, dizziness, nausea, etc.) These symptoms are, however, usually accompanied by extreme fear, particularly the fear of dying. Like adults with Panic Disorder, children may attempt to avoid any situation they feel is a "trigger" for their attacks.

Specific Phobia

A specific phobia is any kind of anxiety disorder that amounts to an unreasonable or irrational fear related to exposure to specific objects or situations. As a result, the affected person tends to avoid contact with the objects or situations and, in severe cases, any mention or depiction of them. The fear can, in fact, be disabling to their daily lives.

The fear or anxiety may be triggered both by the presence and the anticipation of the specific object or situation. A person who encounters that of which they are phobic will often show signs of fear or express discomfort. In some cases, it can result in a panic attack. In most adults, the person may logically know the fear is unreasonable but still find it difficult to control the anxiety. Thus, this condition may significantly impair the person's functioning and even physical health.

Specific phobia affects up to 12% of people at some point in their life.

Diagnosis

Main features of diagnostic criteria for specific phobia in the DSM-IV-TR:

- Marked and persistent fear that is excessive or unreasonable, cued by the presence or anticipation of a specific object or situation (e.g., flying, heights, animals, receiving an injection, seeing blood).

- Exposure to the phobic stimulus almost invariably provokes an immediate anxiety response, which may take the form of a situationally bound or situationally predisposed panic attack. In children, the anxiety may be expressed by crying, tantrums, freezing, or clinging.

- The person recognizes that the fear is excessive or unreasonable. In children, this feature may be absent.

- The phobic situation(s) is avoided or else is endured with intense anxiety or distress.

Specific Phobia – DSM 5 Criteria

- Fear or anxiety about a specific object or situation (In children fear/anxiety can be expressed by crying, tantrums, freezing, or clinging)

- The phobic object or situation almost always provokes immediate fear or anxiety

- The phobic object or situation is avoided or endured with intense fear or anxiety

- The fear or anxiety is out of proportion to the actual danger posed by the specific object or situation and to the sociocultural context

- The fear, anxiety, or avoidance is persistent, typically lasting for 6 months or more

- The fear, anxiety, or avoidance causes clinically significant distress or impairment in social, occupational, or other important areas of functioning

- The disturbance is not better explained by symptoms of another mental disorder, including fear, anxiety, and avoidance of situations associated with panic-like symptoms or other incapacitating symptoms; objects or situations related to obsessions; reminders of traumatic events; separation from home or attachment figures; or social situations

Types

According to the fourth revision of the *Diagnostic and Statistical Manual of Mental Disorders*, phobias can be classified under the following general categories:

- Animal type – Fear of dogs, cats, rats and/or mice, pigs, cows, birds, spiders, or snakes.

- Natural environment type – Fear of water (aquaphobia), heights (acrophobia), lightning and thunderstorms (astraphobia), or aging (gerascophobia).

- Situational type – Fear of small confined spaces (claustrophobia), or the dark (nyctophobia).

- Blood/injection/injury type – this includes fear of medical procedures, including needles and injections (trypanophobia), fear of blood (hemophobia) and fear of getting injured.

- Other – children's fears of loud sounds or costumed characters.

Treatment

The following are two therapies normally used in treating specific phobia:

Cognitive behavioral therapy (CBT), a short term, skills-focused therapy that aims to help people diffuse unhelpful emotional responses by helping people consider them differently or change their behavior, is effective in treating specific phobias. Exposure therapy is a particularly effective form of CBT for specific phobias. Medications to aid CBT have not been as encouraging with the exception of adjunctive D-clycoserine.

In general anxiolytic medication is not seen as helpful in specific phobia but benzodiazepines are sometimes used to help resolve acute episodes; as 2007 data were sparse for efficacy of any drug.

Epidemiology

Specific phobias have a one-year prevalence of 8.7% in the USA with 21.9% of the cases being severe, 30.0% moderate and 48.1% mild. The usual age of onset is childhood to adolescence. Women are twice as likely to suffer from specific phobias as men.

Evolutionary theory argues that infants or children develop specific phobias to things that could possibly harm them, so their phobias alert them to the danger. The most common co-occurring disorder for children with a specific phobia is another anxiety disorder. Although comorbidity is frequent for children with specific phobias, it tends to be lower than for other anxiety disorders. Onset is typically between 7 and 9 years of age. Specific phobias can occur at any age but seem to peak between 10 and 13 years of age.

Panic disorder

Panic disorder is an anxiety disorder characterized by recurrent unexpected panic attacks. Panic attacks are sudden periods of intense fear that may include palpitations, sweating, shaking, shortness of breath, numbness, or a feeling that something really bad is going to happen. The maximum degree of symptoms occurs within minutes. There may be ongoing worries about having further attacks and avoidance of places where attacks have occurred in the past.

The cause of panic disorder is unknown. Panic disorder often runs in families. Risk factors include smoking, psychological stress, and a history of child abuse. Diagnosis involves ruling out other potential causes of anxiety including other mental disorders, medical conditions such as heart disease or hyperthyroidism, and drug use. Screening for the condition may be done using a questionnaire.

Panic disorder is usually treated with counselling and medications. The type of counselling used is typically cognitive behavioral therapy (CBT) which is effective in more than half of people. Medications used include antidepressants and occasionally benzodiazepines or beta blockers. Following stopping treatment up to 30% of people have a recurrence.

Panic disorder affects about 2.5% of people at some point in their life. It usually begins during adolescence or early adulthood but any age can be affected. It is less common in children and older people. Women are more often affected than men.

Signs and Symptoms

Panic disorder sufferers usually have a series of intense episodes of extreme anxiety during panic attacks. These attacks typically last about ten minutes, and can be as short-lived as 1–5 minutes, but can last twenty minutes to more than an hour, or until helpful intervention is made. Panic attacks can wax and wane for a period of hours (panic attacks rolling into one another), and the intensity and specific symptoms of panic may vary over the duration.

In some cases, the attack may continue at unabated high intensity, or seem to be increasing in severity. Common symptoms of an attack include rapid heartbeat, perspiration, dizziness, dyspnea, trembling, uncontrollable fear such as: the fear of losing control and going crazy, the fear of dying and hyperventilation. Other symptoms are sweating, a sensation of choking, paralysis, chest pain, nausea, numbness or tingling, chills or hot flashes, faintness, crying and some sense of altered reality. In addition, the person usually has thoughts of impending doom. Individuals suffering from an episode have often a strong wish of escaping from the situation that provoked the attack. The anxiety of panic disorder is particularly severe and noticeably episodic compared to that from generalized anxiety disorder. Panic attacks may be provoked by exposure to certain stimuli (e.g., seeing a mouse) or settings (e.g., the dentist's office). Other attacks may appear unprovoked. Some individuals deal with these events on a regular basis, sometimes daily or weekly. The outward symptoms of a panic attack often cause negative social experiences (e.g., embarrassment, social stigma, social isolation, etc.).

Limited symptom attacks are similar to panic attacks, but have fewer symptoms. Most people with PD experience both panic attacks and limited symptom attacks.

Causes

Psychological Models

While there is not just one explanation for the cause of panic disorder, there are certain perspectives researchers use to explain the disorder. The first one is the biological perspective. Past research concluded that there is irregular norepinephrine activity in people who have panic attacks. Current research also supports this perspective as it has been found that those with panic disorder also have a brain circuit that performs improperly. This circuit consists of the amygdala, central gray matter, ventromedial nucleus of the hypothalamus, and the locus ceruleus.

There is also the cognitive perspective. Theorists believe that people with panic disorder may experience panic reactions because they mistake their bodily sensations for life-threatening situations. These bodily sensations cause some people to feel as though are out of control which may lead to feelings of panic. This misconception of bodily sensations is referred to as anxiety sensitivity and studies suggest that the people who score higher on anxiety sensitivity surveys than other people, are fives times more likely to be diagnosed with panic disorder.

Panic disorder has been found to run in families, and suggests that inheritance plays a strong role in determining who will get it.

Psychological factors, stressful life events, life transitions, and environment as well as often thinking in a way that exaggerates relatively normal bodily reactions are also believed to play a role in the onset of panic disorder. Often the first attacks are triggered by physical illnesses, major stress, or certain medications. People who tend to take on excessive responsibilities may develop a tendency to suffer panic attacks. Post-traumatic stress disorder (PTSD) patients also show a much higher rate of panic disorder than the general population.

Prepulse inhibition has been found to be reduced in patients with panic disorder.

Substance Misuse

Substance abuse is often correlated with panic attacks. The majority of individuals participating in a study determined (63%) of those abusing alcohol reported that alcohol use began prior to the onset of panic, and the majority (59%) of those abusing illicit drugs reported that drug use began first. The study that was conducted documented the panic-substance abuse relationship. Substance abuse began prior to onset of panic and substances were used to self-medicate for panic attacks by only a few subjects.

In another study, 100 methamphetamine-dependent individuals were analyzed for co-morbid psychiatric disorders; of the 100 individuals, 36% were categorized as having co-morbid psychiatric disorders. Mood and Psychotic disorders were more prevalent than anxiety disorders, which accounted for 7% of the 100 sampled individuals.

Smoking

Tobacco smoking increases the risk of developing panic disorder with or without agoraphobia and panic attacks; smoking started in adolescence or early adulthood particularly increases this risk of developing panic disorder. While the mechanism of how smoking increases panic attacks is not fully understood, a few hypotheses have been derived. Smoking cigarettes may lead to panic attacks by causing changes in respiratory function (e.g. feeling short of breath). These respiratory changes in turn can lead to the formation of panic attacks, as respiratory symptoms are a prominent feature of panic. Respiratory abnormalities have been found in children with high levels of anxiety, which suggests that a person with these difficulties may be susceptible to panic attacks, and thus more likely to subsequently develop panic disorder. Nicotine, a stimulant, could contribute to panic attacks. However, nicotine withdrawal may also cause significant anxiety which could contribute to panic attacks.

It is also possible that panic disorder patients smoke cigarettes as a form of self-medication to lessen anxiety. Nicotine and other psychoactive compounds with antidepressant properties in tobacco smoke which act as monoamine oxidase inhibitors in the brain can alter mood and have a calming effect, depending on dose.

Stimulants

A number of clinical studies have shown a positive association between caffeine ingestion and panic disorder and/or anxiogenic effects. People who have panic disorder are more sensitive to the anxiety-provoking effects of caffeine. One of the major anxiety-provoking effects of caffeine is an increase in heart rate.

Certain cold and flu medications containing decongestants may also contain pseudoephedrine, ephedrine, phenylephrine, naphazoline and oxymetazoline. These may be avoided by the use of decongestants formulated to prevent causing high blood pressure.

Alcohol and Sedatives

About 30% of people with panic disorder use alcohol and 17% use other psychoactive drugs. This is in comparison with 61% (alcohol) and 7.9% (other psychoactive drugs) of the general population who use alcohol and psychoactive drugs, respectively. Utilization of recreational drugs or alcohol generally make symptoms worse. Most stimulant drugs (caffeine, nicotine, cocaine) would be expected to worsen the condition, since they directly increase the symptoms of panic, such as heart rate.

Deacon and Valentiner (2000) conducted a study that examined co-morbid panic attacks and substance use in a non-clinical sample of young adults who experienced regular panic attacks. The authors found that compared to healthy controls, therapeutic alcohol and sedative use was greater for non-clinical participants who experienced panic attacks. These findings are consistent with the suggestion made by Cox, Norton, Dorward, and Fergusson (1989) that panic disorder patients self-medicate if they believe that certain substances will be successful in alleviating their symptoms. If panic disorder patients are indeed self-medicating, there may be a portion of the population with undiagnosed panic disorder who will not seek professional help as a result of their own self-medication. In fact, for some patients panic disorder is only diagnosed after they seek treatment for their self-medication habit.

While alcohol initially helps ease panic disorder symptoms, medium- or long-term alcohol abuse can cause panic disorder to develop or worsen during alcohol intoxication, especially during alcohol withdrawal syndrome. This effect is not unique to alcohol but can also occur with long-term use of drugs which have a similar mechanism of action to alcohol such as the benzodiazepines which are sometimes prescribed as tranquilizers to people with alcohol problems. The reason chronic alcohol misuse worsens panic disorder is due to distortion of the brain chemistry and function.

Approximately 10% of patients will experience notable protracted withdrawal symptoms, which can include panic disorder, after discontinuation of benzodiazepines. Protracted withdrawal symptoms tend to resemble those seen during the first couple of months of withdrawal but usually are of a subacute level of severity compared to the symptoms seen during the first 2 or 3 months of withdrawal. It is not known definitively whether such symptoms persisting long after withdrawal are related to true pharmacological withdrawal or whether they are due to structural neuronal damage as result of chronic use of benzodiazepines or withdrawal. Nevertheless, such symptoms do typically lessen as the months and years go by eventually disappearing altogether.

A significant proportion of patients attending mental health services for conditions including anxiety disorders such as panic disorder or social phobia have developed these conditions as a result of alcohol or sedative abuse. Anxiety may pre-exist alcohol or sedative independence, which then acts to perpetuate or worsen the underlying anxiety disorder. Someone suffering the toxic effects of alcohol abuse or chronic sedative use or abuse will not benefit from other therapies or medications for underlying psychiatric conditions. as they do not address the root cause of the symptoms. Recovery from sedative symptoms may temporarily worsen during alcohol withdrawal or benzodiazepine withdrawal.

Mechanism

There are other researchers studying some individuals with panic disorder and propose they may have a chemical imbalance within the limbic system and one of its regulatory chemicals GABA-A. The reduced production of GABA-A sends false information to the amygdala which regulates the body's "fight or flight" response mechanism and, in return, produces the physiological symptoms that lead to the disorder. Clonazepam, an anticonvulsant benzodiazepine with a long half-life, has been successful in keeping the condition under control.

Recently, researchers have begun to identify mediators and moderators of aspects of panic disorder. One such mediator is the partial pressure of carbon dioxide, which mediates the relationship between panic disorder patients receiving breathing training and anxiety sensitivity; thus, breathing training affects the partial pressure of carbon dioxide in a patient's arterial blood, which in turn lowers anxiety sensitivity. Another mediator is hypochondriacal concerns, which mediate the relationship between anxiety sensitivity and panic symptomatology; thus, anxiety sensitivity affects hypochondriacal concerns which, in turn, affect panic symptomatology.

Perceived threat control has been identified as a moderator within panic disorder, moderating the relationship between anxiety sensitivity and agoraphobia; thus, the level of perceived threat control dictates the degree to which anxiety sensitivity results in agoraphobia. Another recently identified moderator of panic disorder is genetic variations in the gene coding for galanin; these genetic variations moderate the relationship between females suffering from panic disorder and the level of severity of panic disorder symptomatology.

Diagnosis

The DSM-IV-TR diagnostic criteria for panic disorder require unexpected, recurrent panic attacks, followed in at least one instance by at least a month of a significant and related behavior change, a persistent concern of more attacks, or a worry about the attack's consequences. There are two types, one with and one without agoraphobia. Diagnosis is excluded by attacks due to a drug or medical condition, or by panic attacks that are better accounted for by other mental disorders. The ICD-10 diagnostic criteria:

The essential feature is recurrent attacks of severe anxiety (panic), which are not restricted to any particular situation or set of circumstances and are therefore unpredictable. The dominant symptoms include:

- sudden onset of palpitations
- chest pain
- choking sensations
- dizziness
- feelings of unreality (depersonalization or derealization)
- secondary fear of dying, losing control, or going mad

Panic disorder should not be given as the main diagnosis if the patient has a depressive disorder at the time the attacks start; in these circumstances, the panic attacks are probably secondary to depression.

Treatment

Panic disorder is a serious health problem that in many cases can be successfully treated, although there is no known cure. Identification of treatments that engender as full a response as possible, and can minimize relapse, is imperative. Cognitive behavioural therapy and positive self-talk specific for panic are the treatment of choice for panic disorder. Several studies show that 85 to 90 percent of panic disorder patients treated with CBT recover completely from their panic attacks within 12 weeks. When cognitive behavioral therapy is not an option, pharmacotherapy can be used. SSRIs are considered a first-line pharmacotherapeutic option.

Psychotherapy

Panic disorder is not the same as phobic symptoms, although phobias commonly result from panic disorder. CBT and one tested form of psychodynamic psychotherapy have been shown efficacious in treating panic disorder with and without agoraphobia. A number of randomized clinical trials have shown that CBT achieves reported panic-free status in 70–90% of patients about 2 years after treatment.

Clinically, a combination of psychotherapy and medication can often produce good results, although research evidence of this approach has been less robust. Some improvement may be noticed in a fairly short period of time, about 6 to 8 weeks. Psychotherapy can improve the effectiveness of medication, reduce the likelihood of relapse for someone who has discontinued medication, and offer help for people with panic disorder who do not respond at all to medication.

The goal of cognitive behavior therapy is to help a patient reorganize thinking processes and anxious thoughts regarding an experience that provokes panic. An approach that proved successful for 87% of patients in a controlled trial is interoceptive therapy, which simulates the symptoms of panic to allow patients to experience them in a controlled environment.

Symptom inductions generally occur for *one minute* and may include:

- Intentional hyperventilation – creates lightheadedness, derealization, blurred vision, dizziness

- Spinning in a chair – creates dizziness, disorientation

- Straw breathing – creates dyspnea, airway constriction

- Breath holding – creates sensation of being out of breath

- Running in place – creates increased heart rate, respiration, perspiration

- Body tensing – creates feelings of being tense and vigilant

The key to the induction is that the exercises should mimic the most frightening symptoms of a panic attack. Symptom inductions should be repeated three to five times per day until the patient has little to no anxiety in relation to the symptoms that were induced. Often it will take a period of weeks for the afflicted to feel no anxiety in relation to the induced symptoms. With repeated trials, a person learns through experience that these internal sensations do not need to be feared and becomes less sensitized or desensitized to the internal sensation. After repeated trials, when nothing catastrophic happens, the brain learns (hippocampus and amygdala) to not fear the sensations, and the sympathetic nervous system activation fades. However, in real-life situations panic may escalate independently of whether the subject is fearful of the minor symptoms associated with panic. The subject may have no fear of fast heart rate, hyperventilation or derealization, but may nevertheless feel terror, and it is the terror that may cause the other symptoms.

For patients whose panic disorder involves agoraphobia, the traditional cognitive therapy approach has been in vivo exposure, in which the affected individual, accompanied by a therapist, is gradually exposed to the actual situation that provokes panic.

Another form of psychotherapy which has shown effectiveness in controlled clinical trials is panic-focused psychodynamic psychotherapy, which focuses on the role of dependency, separation anxiety, and anger in causing panic disorder. The underlying theory posits that due to biochemical vulnerability, traumatic early experiences, or both, people with panic disorder have a fearful dependence on others for their sense of security, which leads to separation anxiety and defensive anger. Therapy involves first exploring the stressors that lead to panic episodes, then probing the psychodynamics of the conflicts underlying panic disorder and the defense mechanisms that contribute to the attacks, with attention to transference and separation anxiety issues implicated in the therapist-patient relationship.

Comparative clinical studies suggest that muscle relaxation techniques and breathing exercises are not efficacious in reducing panic attacks. In fact, breathing exercises may actually increase the risk of relapse.

Appropriate treatment by an experienced professional can prevent panic attacks or at least substantially reduce their severity and frequency — bringing significant relief to percent of people with panic disorder. Relapses may occur, but they can often be effectively treated just like the initial episode.

vanApeldoorn, F.J. et al. (2011) demonstrated the additive value of a combined treatment incorporating an SSRI treatment intervention with cognitive behavior therapy (CBT). Gloster et al. (2011) went on to examine the role of the therapist in CBT. They randomized patients into two groups: one being treated with CBT in a therapist guided environment, and the second receiving CBT through instruction only, with no therapist guided sessions. The findings indicated that the first group had a somewhat better response rate, but that both groups demonstrated a significant improvement in reduction of panic symptomatology. These findings lend credibility to the application of CBT programs to patients who are unable to access therapeutic services due to financial, or geographic inaccessibility. Koszycky et al. (2011) discuss the efficacy of self-administered cognitive behavioural therapy (SCBT) in situations where patients are unable to retain the services of a therapist. Their study demonstrates that it is possible for SCBT in combination with an SSRI to be as effective as therapist-guided CBT with SSRI. Each of these studies contributes to a new avenue of research that allows effective treatment interventions to be made more easily accessible to the population.

Cognitive Behavioral Therapy

Cognitive behavioral therapy encourages patients to confront the triggers that induce arouse their anxiety. By facing the very cause of the anxiety, it is thought to help diminish the irrational fears that are causing the issues to begin with. The therapy begins with calming breathing exercises, followed by noting the changes in physical sensations felt as soon as anxiety begins to enter the body. Many clients are encouraged to keep journals. In other cases, therapists may try and induce feelings of anxiety so that the root of the fear can be identified.

Comorbid clinical depression, personality disorders and alcohol abuse are known risk factors for treatment failure.

As with many disorders, having a support structure of family and friends who understand the condition can help increase the rate of recovery. During an attack, it is not uncommon for the sufferer to develop irrational, immediate fear, which can often be dispelled by a supporter who is familiar with the condition. For more serious or active treatment, there are support groups for anxiety sufferers which can help people understand and deal with the disorder.

Current treatment guidelines American Psychiatric Association and the American Medical Association primarily recommend either cognitive-behavioral therapy or one of a variety of psychopharmacological interventions. Some evidence exists supporting the superiority of combined treatment approaches.

Another option is self-help based on principles of cognitive-behavioral therapy. Using a book or a website, a person does the kinds of exercises that would be used in therapy, but they do it on their own, perhaps with some email or phone support from a therapist. A systematic analysis of trials testing this kind of self-help found that websites, books, and other materials based on cognitive-behavioral therapy could help some people. The best-studied conditions are panic disorder and social phobia.

Medication

Appropriate medications are effective for panic disorder. Selective serotonin reuptake inhibitors are first line treatments rather than benzodiazapines due to concerns with the latter regarding tolerance, dependence and abuse. Although there is little evidence that pharmacological interventions can directly alter phobias, few studies have been performed, and medication treatment of panic makes phobia treatment far easier (an example in Europe where only 8% of patients receive appropriate treatment). Medications can include:

- Antidepressants (SSRIs, MAOIs, tricyclic antidepressants and norepinephrine reuptake inhibitors): these are taken regularly every day, and alter neurotransmitter configurations which in turn can help to block symptoms. Although these medications are described as "antidepressants", nearly all of them — especially the tricyclic antidepressants — have anti-anxiety properties, in part, due to their sedative effects. SSRIs have been known to exacerbate symptoms in panic disorder patients, especially in the beginning of treatment and have even provoked panic attacks in otherwise healthy individuals. SSRIs are also known to produce withdrawal symptoms which include rebound anxiety and panic attacks. Comorbid depression has been cited as imparting the worst course, leading to chronic, disabling illness.

- Antianxiety agents (benzodiazepines): Use of benzodiazepines for panic disorder is controversial with opinion differing in the medical literature. The American Psychiatric Association states that benzodiazepines can be effective for the treatment of panic disorder and recommends that the choice of whether to use benzodiazepines, antidepressants with anti-panic properties or psychotherapy should be based on the individual patient's history and characteristics. Other experts believe that benzodiazepines are best avoided due to the risks of the development of tolerance and physical dependence. The World Federation of Societies of Biological Psychiatry, say that benzodiazepines should not be used as a first-line treatment option but are an option for treatment-resistant cases of panic disorder. Despite increasing focus on the use of antidepressants and other agents for the treatment of anxiety as recommended best practice, benzodiazepines have remained a commonly used medication for panic disorder. They reported that in their view there is insufficient evidence to recommend one treatment over another for panic disorder. The APA noted that while benzodiazepines have the advantage of a rapid onset of action, that this is offset by the risk of developing a benzodiazepine dependence. The National Institute of Clinical Excellence came to a different conclusion, they pointed out the problems of using uncontrolled clinical trials to assess the effectiveness of pharmacotherapy and based on placebo-controlled research they concluded that benzodiazepines were not effective in the long-term for panic disorder and recommended that benzodiazepines not be used for longer than 4 weeks for panic disorder. Instead NICE clinical guidelines recommend alternative pharmacotherapeutic or psychotherapeutic interventions.

Other Treatments

For some people, anxiety can be greatly reduced by discontinuing the use of caffeine. Anxiety can temporarily increase during caffeine withdrawal.

Epidemiology

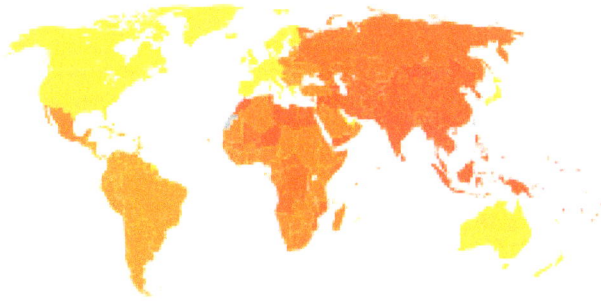

Age-standardized disability-adjusted life year rates for panic disorder per 100,000 inhabitants in 2004.

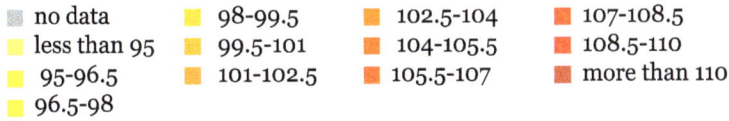

no data	98-99.5	102.5-104	107-108.5
less than 95	99.5-101	104-105.5	108.5-110
95-96.5	101-102.5	105.5-107	more than 110
96.5-98			

Panic disorder typically begins during early adulthood; roughly half of all people who have panic disorder develop the condition before age 24, especially those subjected to traumatic experiences. However, some sources say that the majority of young people affected for the first time are between the ages of 25 and 30. Women are twice as likely as men to develop panic disorder and it occurs more often in people with above average intelligence.

Panic disorder can continue for months or years, depending on how and when treatment is sought. If left untreated, it may worsen to the point where one's life is seriously affected by panic attacks and by attempts to avoid or conceal the condition. In fact, many people have had problems with personal relationships or employment while struggling to cope with panic disorder. Some people with panic disorder may conceal their condition because of the stigma of mental illness. In some individuals, symptoms may occur frequently for a period of months or years, then many years may pass without symptoms. In some cases, the symptoms persist at the same level indefinitely. There is also some evidence that many individuals (especially those who develop symptoms at an early age) may experience symptom cessation later in life (e.g. past age 50).

In 2000, the World Health Organization found prevalence and incidence rates for panic disorder to be very similar across the globe. Age-standardized prevalence per 100,000 ranged from 309 in Africa to 330 in East Asia for men and from 613 in Africa to 649 in North America, Oceania, and Europe for women.

Children

A retrospective study has shown that 40% of adult panic disorder patients reported that their disorder began before the age of 20. In an article examining the phenomenon of panic disorder in youth, Diler et al. (2004) found that only a few past studies have examined the occurrence of juvenile panic disorder. They report that these studies have found that the symptoms of juvenile panic disorder almost replicate those found in adults (e.g. heart palpitations, sweating, trembling, hot flashes, nausea, abdominal distress, and chills). The anxiety disorders co-exist with staggeringly high numbers of other mental disorders in adults. The same comorbid disorders that are seen in adults are also reported in children with juvenile panic disorder. Last and Strauss (1989) examined a sample of 17 adolescents with panic disorder and found high rates of comorbid anxiety disorders, major depressive disorder, and conduct disorders. Eassau et al. (1999) also found a high number of comorbid disorders in a community-based sample of adolescents with panic attacks or juvenile panic disorder. Within the sample, adolescents were found to have the following comorbid disorders: major depressive disorder (80%), dysthymic disorder (40%), generalized anxiety disorder (40%), somatoform disorders (40%), substance abuse (40%), and specific phobia (20%). Consistent with this previous work, Diler et al. (2004) found similar results in their study in which 42 youths with juvenile panic disorder were examined. Compared to non-panic anxiety disordered youths, children with panic disorder had higher rates of comorbid major depressive disorder and bipolar disorder.

Children differ from adolescents and adults in their interpretation and ability to express their experience. Like adults, children experience physical symptoms including accelerated heart rate, sweating, trembling or shaking, shortness of breath, nausea or stomach pain, dizziness or light-headedness. In addition, children also experience cognitive symptoms like fear of dying, feelings of being detached from oneself, feelings of losing control or going crazy, but they are unable to vocalize these higher order manifestations of fear. They simply know that something is going wrong and that they are very afraid. Children can only describe the physical symptoms. They have not yet developed the constructs to put these symptoms together and label them as fear. Parents often feel helpless when they watch a child suffer. They can help children give a name to their experience, and empower them to overcome the fear they are experiencing

The role of the parent in treatment and intervention for children diagnosed with panic disorder is discussed by McKay & Starch (2011). They point out that there are several levels at which parental involvement should be considered. The first involves the initial assessment. Parents, as well as the child, should be screened for attitudes and treatment goals, as well as for levels of anxiety or conflict in the home. The second involves the treatment process in which the therapist should meet with the family as a unit as frequently as possible. Ideally, all family members should be aware and trained in the process of cognitive behavior therapy (CBT) in order to encourage the child to rationalize and face fears rather than employ avoidant safety behaviors. McKay & Storch (2011) suggest training/modeling of therapeutic techniques and in session involvement of the parents in the treatment of children to enhance treatment efficacy.

Despite the evidence pointing to the existence of early-onset panic disorder, the DSM-IV-TR currently only recognizes six anxiety disorders in children: separation anxiety disorder, generalized anxiety disorder, specific phobia, obsessive-compulsive disorder, social anxiety disorder (a.k.a. social phobia), and post-traumatic stress disorder. Panic disorder is notably excluded from this list.

Agoraphobia

Agoraphobia is an anxiety disorder characterized by symptoms of anxiety in situations where the person perceives the environment to be unsafe with no easy way to get away. These situations can include open spaces, public transit, shopping malls, or simply being outside the home. Being in these situations may result in a panic attack. The symptoms occur nearly every time the situation is encountered and last for more than six months. Those affected will go to great lengths to avoid these situations. In severe cases people may become unable to leave their homes.

Agoraphobia is believed to be due to a combination of genetic and environmental factors. The condition often runs in families, and stressful events such as the death of a parent or being attacked may be a trigger. In the DSM-5 agoraphobia is classified as a phobia along with specific phobias and social phobia. Other conditions that can produce similar symptoms include separation anxiety, posttraumatic stress disorder, and major depressive disorder. Those affected are at higher risk of depression and substance use disorder.

Without treatment it is uncommon for agoraphobia to resolve. Treatment is typically with a type of counselling called cognitive behavioral therapy (CBT). CBT results in resolution for about half of people. Agoraphobia affects about 1.7% of adults. Women are affected about twice as often as men. The condition often begins in early adulthood and becomes less common in old age. It is rare in children.

Signs and Symptoms

Agoraphobia is a condition where sufferers become anxious in unfamiliar environments or where they perceive that they have little control. Triggers for this anxiety may include wide-open spaces, crowds (social anxiety), or traveling (even short distances). Agoraphobia is often, but not always, compounded by a fear of social embarrassment, as the agoraphobic fears the onset of a panic attack and appearing distraught in public. Most of the time they avoid these areas and stay in the comfort of their safe haven. This is also sometimes called "social agoraphobia", which may be a subtype of social anxiety disorder.

Agoraphobia is also defined as "a fear, sometimes terrifying, by those who have experienced one or more panic attacks". In these cases, the sufferer is fearful of a particular place because they have experienced a panic attack at the same location at a previous time. Fearing the onset of another panic attack, the sufferer is fearful or even avoids a location. Some refuse to leave their homes even in medical emergencies because the fear of being outside of their comfort areas is too great.

The sufferers can sometimes go to great lengths to avoid the locations where they have experienced the onset of a panic attack. Agoraphobia, as described in this manner, is actually a symptom professionals check when making a diagnosis of panic disorder.

Other syndromes like obsessive compulsive disorder or post-traumatic stress disorder can also cause agoraphobia. Essentially, any irrational fear that keeps one from going outside can cause the syndrome.

Agoraphobics may suffer from temporary separation anxiety disorder when certain other individuals of the household depart from the residence temporarily, such as a parent or spouse, or when the agoraphobic is left home alone. Such temporary conditions can result in an increase in anxiety or a panic attack or feeling the need to separate themselves from family or maybe friends.

Another common associative disorder of agoraphobia is thanatophobia, the fear of death. The anxiety level of agoraphobics often increases when dwelling upon the idea of eventually dying, which they may consciously or unconsciously associate with being the ultimate separation from their emotional comfort and safety zones and loved ones, even for those who may otherwise believe in some form of afterlife.

Panic Attacks

Agoraphobia patients can experience sudden panic attacks when traveling to places where they fear they are out of control, help would be difficult to obtain, or they could be embarrassed. During a panic attack, epinephrine is released in large amounts, triggering the body's natural fight-or-flight response. A panic attack typically has an abrupt onset, building to maximum intensity within 10 to 15 minutes, and rarely lasts longer than 30 minutes. Symptoms of a panic attack include palpitations, rapid heartbeat, sweating, trembling, nausea, vomiting, dizziness, tightness in the throat, and shortness of breath. Many patients report a fear of dying or of losing control of emotions and/or behaviors.

Causes

Although the exact causes of agoraphobia are unknown, some clinicians who have treated or attempted to treat agoraphobia offer plausible hypotheses. The condition has been linked to the presence of other anxiety disorders, a stressful environment, or substance abuse.

Research has uncovered a link between agoraphobia and difficulties with spatial orientation. Individuals without agoraphobia are able to maintain balance by combining information from their vestibular system, their visual system, and their proprioceptive sense. A disproportionate number of agoraphobics have weak vestibular function and consequently rely more on visual or tactile signals. They may become disoriented when visual cues are sparse (as in wide-open spaces) or overwhelming (as in crowds). Likewise, they may be confused by sloping or irregular surfaces. In a virtual reality study, agoraphobics showed impaired processing of changing audiovisual data in comparison with nonsuffering subjects.

Substance Induced

Chronic use of tranquilizers and sleeping pills such as benzodiazepines has been linked to onset of agoraphobia. In 10 patients who had developed agoraphobia during benzodiazepine dependence, symptoms abated within the first year of assisted withdrawal. Similarly, alcohol use disorders are associated with panic with or without agoraphobia; this association may be due to the long-term effects of alcohol misuse causing a distortion in brain chemistry. Tobacco smoking has also been associated with the development and emergence of agoraphobia, often with panic disorder; it is uncertain how tobacco smoking results in anxiety-panic with or without agoraphobia symptoms, but the direct effects of nicotine dependence or the effects of tobacco smoke on breathing have been suggested as possible causes. Self-medication or a combination of factors may also explain the association between tobacco smoking and agoraphobia and panic.

Attachment Theory

Some scholars have explained agoraphobia as an attachment deficit, i.e., the temporary loss of the ability to tolerate spatial separations from a secure base. Recent empirical research has also linked attachment and spatial theories of agoraphobia.

Spatial Theory

In the social sciences, a perceived clinical bias exists in agoraphobia research. Branches of the social sciences, especially geography, have increasingly become interested in what may be thought of as a spatial phenomenon. One such approach links the development of agoraphobia with modernity. Factors considered contributing to agoraphobia within modernity are the ubiquity of cars and urbanization. These have helped develop the expansion of public space, on one hand, and the contraction of private space on the other, thus creating in the minds of agoraphobic-prone people a tense, unbridgeable gulf between the two.

Evolutionary Psychology

An evolutionary psychology view is that the more unusual primary agoraphobia without panic attacks may be due to a different mechanism from agoraphobia with panic attacks. Primary agoraphobia without panic attacks may be a specific phobia explained by it once having been evolutionarily advantageous to avoid exposed, large, open spaces without cover or concealment. Agoraphobia with panic attack, though, may be an avoidance response secondary to the panic attacks due to fear of the situations in which the panic attacks occurred.

Diagnosis

Most people who present to mental health specialists develop agoraphobia after the onset of panic disorder. Agoraphobia is best understood as an adverse behavioral outcome of repeated panic attacks and subsequent anxiety and preoccupation with these attacks that leads to an avoidance of situations where a panic attack could occur. Early treatment of panic disorder can often prevent agoraphobia. Agoraphobia is typically determined when symptoms are worse than panic disorder, but also do not meet the criteria for other anxiety disorders such as depression. In rare cases where agoraphobics do not meet the criteria used to diagnose panic disorder, the formal diagnosis of agoraphobia without history of panic disorder is used (primary agoraphobia).

Treatments

Therapy

Systematic desensitization can provide lasting relief to the majority of patients with panic disorder and agoraphobia. Disappearance of residual and subclinical agoraphobic avoidance, and not simply of panic attacks, should be the aim of exposure therapy. Similarly, systematic desensitization may also be used. Many patients can deal with exposure easier if they are in the company of a friend on whom they can rely. Patients must remain in the situation until anxiety has abated, because if they leave the situation, the phobic response will not decrease and it may even rise.

A related exposure treatment is *in vivo* exposure, a Cognitive Behavioral Therapy method, that gradually exposes patients to the feared situations or objects. This treatment was largely effective with an effect size from $d = 0.78$ to $d = 1.34$, and these effects were shown to increase over time, proving that the treatment had long term efficacy (up to 12 months after treatment).

Psychological interventions in combination with pharmaceutical treatments were overall more effective than treatments simply involving either CBT or pharmaceuticals. Further research showed there was no significant effect between using group CBT versus individual CBT.

Cognitive restructuring has also proved useful in treating agoraphobia. This treatment involves coaching a participant through a dianoetic discussion, with the intent of replacing irrational, counterproductive beliefs with more factual and beneficial ones.

Relaxation techniques are often useful skills for the agoraphobic to develop, as they can be used to stop or prevent symptoms of anxiety and panic.

Medications

Antidepressant medications most commonly used to treat anxiety disorders are mainly selective serotonin reuptake inhibitors. Benzodiazepines, monoamine oxidase inhibitor, and tricyclic antidepressants are also sometimes prescribed for treatment of agoraphobia. Antidepressants are important because some have antipanic effects. Antidepressants should be used in conjunction with exposure as a form of self-help or with cognitive behaviour therapy. A combination of medication and cognitive behaviour therapy is sometimes the most effective treatment for agoraphobia.

Benzodiazepines, antianxiety medications such as alprazolam and clonazepam, are used to treat anxiety and can also help control the symptoms of a panic attack. If taken in doses larger than those prescribed, or for too long, they can cause dependence. Side effects may include confusion, drowsiness, light-headedness, loss of balance, and memory loss.

Alternative Medicine

Eye movement desensitization and reprocessing (EMDR) has been studied as a possible treatment for agoraphobia, with poor results. As such, EMDR is only recommended in cases where cognitive-behavioral approaches have proven ineffective or in cases where agoraphobia has developed following trauma.

Many people with anxiety disorders benefit from joining a self-help or support group (telephone conference-call support groups or online support groups being of particular help for completely housebound individuals). Sharing problems and achievements with others, as well as sharing various self-help tools, are common activities in these groups. In particular, stress management techniques and various kinds of meditation practices and visualization techniques can help people with anxiety disorders calm themselves and may enhance the effects of therapy, as can service to others, which can distract from the self-absorption that tends to go with anxiety problems. Also, preliminary evidence suggests aerobic exercise may have a calming effect. Since caffeine, certain illicit drugs, and even some over-the-counter cold medications can aggravate the symptoms of anxiety disorders, they should be avoided.

Epidemiology

Agoraphobia occurs about twice as commonly among women as it does in men. The gender difference may be attributable to several factors: sociocultural traditions that encourage, or permit, the greater expression of avoidance coping strategies by women (including dependent and helpless behaviors), women perhaps being more likely to seek help and therefore be diagnosed, and men being more likely to abuse alcohol in reaction to anxiety and be diagnosed as an alcoholic. Research has not yet produced a single clear explanation for the gender difference in agoraphobia.

Panic disorder with or without agoraphobia affects roughly 5.1% of Americans, and about 1/3 of this population with panic disorder have comorbid agoraphobia. It is uncommon to have agoraphobia without panic attacks, with only 0.17% of people with agorophobia not presenting panic disorders as well.

Social Anxiety Disorder

Social anxiety disorder (SAD), also known as social phobia, is an anxiety disorder characterized by a significant amount of fear in one or more social situations, causing considerable distress and impaired ability to function in at least some parts of daily life. These fears can be triggered by perceived or actual scrutiny from others.

Physical symptoms often include excessive blushing, excess sweating, trembling, palpitations, and nausea. Stammering may be present, along with rapid speech. Panic attacks can also occur under intense fear and discomfort. Some sufferers may use alcohol or other drugs to reduce fears and inhibitions at social events. It is common for sufferers of social phobia to self-medicate in this fashion, especially if they are undiagnosed, untreated, or both; this can lead to alcoholism, eating disorders or other kinds of substance abuse. SAD is sometimes referred to as an *illness of lost opportunities* where "individuals make major life choices to accommodate their illness". According to ICD-10 guidelines, the main diagnostic criteria of social phobia are fear of being the focus of attention, or fear of behaving in a way that will be embarrassing or humiliating, avoidance and anxiety symptoms. Standardized rating scales can be used to screen for social anxiety disorder and measure the severity of anxiety.

The first line treatment for social anxiety disorder is cognitive behavioral therapy (CBT) with medications recommended only in those who are not interested in therapy. CBT is effective in treating social phobia, whether delivered individually or in a group setting. The cognitive and behavioral components seek to change thought patterns and physical reactions to anxiety-inducing situations. The attention given to social anxiety disorder has significantly increased since 1999 with the approval and marketing of drugs for its treatment. Prescribed medications include several classes of antidepressants: selective serotonin reuptake inhibitors (SSRIs), serotonin-norepinephrine reuptake inhibitors (SNRIs), and monoamine oxidase inhibitors (MAOIs). Other commonly used medications include beta blockers and benzodiazepines. It is the most common anxiety disorder with up to 10% of people being affected at some point in their life.

Signs and Symptoms

Cognitive Aspects

In cognitive models of social anxiety disorder, those with social phobias experience dread over how they will be presented to others. They may feel overly self-conscious, pay high self-attention after the activity, or have high performance standards for themselves. According to the social psychology theory of self-presentation, a sufferer attempts to create a well-mannered impression towards others but believes he or she is unable to do so. Many times, prior to the potentially anxiety-provoking social situation, sufferers may deliberately review what could go wrong and how to deal with each unexpected case. After the event, they may have the perception that they performed un-satisfactorily. Consequently, they will perceive anything that may have possibly been abnormal as embarrassing. These thoughts may extend for weeks or longer. Cognitive distortions are a hallmark, and are learned about in CBT (cognitive-behavioral thera-py). Thoughts are often self-defeating and inaccurate. Those with social phobia tend to interpret neutral or ambiguous conversations with a negative outlook, and many studies suggest that socially anxious individuals remember more negative memories than those less distressed.

An example of an instance may be that of an employee presenting to their co-work-ers. During the presentation, the person may stutter a word, upon which he or she may worry that other people significantly noticed and think that their perceptions of him or her as a presenter have been tarnished. This cognitive thought propels further anxiety which compounds with further stuttering, sweating, and, potential-ly, a panic attack.

Behavioral Aspects

Social anxiety disorder is a persistent fear of one or more situations in which the person is exposed to possible scrutiny by others and fears that he or she may do something or act in a way that will be humiliating or embarrassing. It exceeds nor-mal "shyness" as it leads to excessive social avoidance and substantial social or occupational impairment. Feared activities may include almost any type of social interaction, especially small groups, dating, parties, talking to strangers, restau-rants, interviews, etc.

Those who suffer from social anxiety disorder fear being judged by others in society. In particular, individuals with social anxiety are nervous in the presence of people with authority and feel uncomfortable during physical examinations. People who suffer from this disorder may behave a certain way or say something and then feel embarrassed or humiliated after. As a result, they often choose to isolate themselves from society to avoid such situations. They may also feel uncomfortable meeting people they do not know, and act distant when they are with large groups of people. In some cases, they may show evidence of this disorder by avoiding eye contact, or blushing when someone is talking to them.

According to psychologist B. F. Skinner, phobias are controlled by escape and avoid-ance behaviors. For instance, a student may leave the room when talking in front of the class (escape) and refrain from doing verbal presentations because of the previously encountered anxiety attack (avoid). Major avoidance behaviors could include an al-most pathological/compulsive lying behavior in order to preserve self-image and avoid judgement in front of others. Minor avoidance behaviors are exposed when a person avoids eye contact and crosses his/her arms to avoid recognizable shaking. A fight-or-flight response is then triggered in such events.

Physiological Aspects

Physiological effects, similar to those in other anxiety disorders, are present in social phobics. In adults, it may be tears as well as excessive sweating, nausea, difficulty breathing, shaking, and palpitations as a result of the fight-or-flight response. The walk disturbance (where a person is so worried about how they walk that they may lose balance) may appear, especially when passing a group of people. Blushing is commonly exhibited by individuals suffering from social phobia. These visible symptoms further reinforce the anxiety in the presence of others. A 2006 study found that the area of the brain called the amygdala, part of the limbic system, is hyperactive when patients are shown threatening faces or confronted with frightening situations. They found that patients with more severe social phobia showed a correlation with the increased response in the amygdala.

Comorbidity

SAD shows a high degree of co-occurrence with other psychiatric disorders. In fact, a population-based study found that 66% of those with SAD had one or more additional mental health disorders. SAD often occurs alongside low self-esteem and most commonly clinical depression, perhaps due to a lack of personal relationships and long periods of isolation related to social avoidance. Clinical depression is 1.49 to 3.5 times more likely to occur in those with SAD. Anxiety disorders are also very common in patients with SAD, in particular generalized anxiety disorder. Avoidant personality disorder is also highly correlated with SAD, with comorbidity rates ranging from 25% to 89%.

To try to reduce their anxiety and alleviate depression, people with social phobia may use alcohol or other drugs, which can lead to substance abuse. It is estimated that one-fifth of patients with social anxiety disorder also suffer from alcohol dependence. However, some research suggests SAD is unrelated to, or even protective against alcohol-related problems. Those who suffer from both alcoholism and social anxiety disorder are more likely to avoid group-based treatments and to relapse compared to people who do not have this combination.

Differential Diagnosis

The DSM-IV criteria stated that an individual cannot receive a diagnosis of social anxiety disorder if their symptoms are better accounted for by one of the autism spectrum disorders such as autism and Asperger syndrome.

Because of its close relationship and overlapping symptoms, treating people with social phobia may help to understand the underlying connections to other mental disorders. Social anxiety disorder is often linked to bipolar disorder and attention deficit hyperactivity disorder (ADHD) and some believe that they share an underlying cyclothymic-anxious-sensitive disposition. The co-occurrence of ADHD and social phobia is very high; especially when SCT symptoms are present.

Causes

Research into the causes of social anxiety and social phobia is wide-ranging, encompassing multiple perspectives from neuroscience to sociology. Scientists have yet to pinpoint the exact causes. Studies suggest that genetics can play a part in combination with environmental factors. Social phobia is not caused by other mental disorders or by substance abuse. Generally, social anxiety begins at a specific point in an individual's life. This will develop over time as the person struggles to recover. Eventually, mild social awkwardness can develop into symptoms of social anxiety or phobia.

Genetics

It has been shown that there is a two to threefold greater risk of having social phobia if a first-degree relative also has the disorder. This could be due to genetics and/or due to children acquiring social fears and avoidance through processes of observational learning or parental psychosocial education. Studies of identical twins brought up (via adoption) in different families have indicated that, if one twin developed social anxiety disorder, then the other was between 30 percent and 50 percent more likely than average to also develop the disorder. To some extent this 'heritability' may not be specific – for example, studies have found that if a parent has any kind of anxiety disorder or clinical depression, then a child is somewhat more likely to develop an anxiety disorder or social phobia. Studies suggest that parents of those with social anxiety disorder tend to be more socially isolated themselves (Bruch and Heimberg, 1994; Caster et al., 1999), and shyness in adoptive parents is significantly correlated with shyness in adopted children (Daniels and Plomin, 1985).

Growing up with overprotective and hypercritical parents has also been associated with social anxiety disorder. Adolescents who were rated as having an insecure (anxious-ambivalent) attachment with their mother as infants were twice as likely to develop anxiety disorders by late adolescence, including social phobia.

A related line of research has investigated 'behavioural inhibition' in infants – early signs of an inhibited and introspective or fearful nature. Studies have shown that around 10–15 percent of individuals show this early temperament, which appears to be partly due to genetics. Some continue to show this trait into adolescence and adulthood, and appear to be more likely to develop social anxiety disorder.

Social Experiences

A previous negative social experience can be a trigger to social phobia, perhaps particularly for individuals high in 'interpersonal sensitivity'. For around half of those diagnosed with social anxiety disorder, a specific traumatic or humiliating social event appears to be associated with the onset or worsening of the disorder; this kind of event appears to be particularly related to specific (performance) social phobia, for example regarding public speaking (Stemberg *et al.*, 1995). As well as direct experiences, observing or hearing about the socially negative experiences of others (e.g. a faux pas committed by someone), or verbal warnings of social problems and dangers, may also make the development of a social anxiety disorder more likely. Social anxiety disorder may be caused by the longer-term effects of not fitting in, or being bullied, rejected or ignored (Beidel and Turner, 1998). Shy adolescents or avoidant adults have emphasised unpleasant experiences with peers or childhood bullying or harassment (Gilmartin, 1987). In one study, popularity was found to be negatively correlated with social anxiety, and children who were neglected by their peers reported higher social anxiety and fear of negative evaluation than other categories of children. Socially phobic children appear less likely to receive positive reactions from peers and anxious or inhibited children may isolate themselves.

Cultural Influences

Cultural factors that have been related to social anxiety disorder include a society's attitude towards shyness and avoidance, affecting the ability to form relationships or access employment or education, and shame. One study found that the effects of parenting are different depending on the culture – American children appear more likely to develop social anxiety disorder if their parents emphasize the importance of others' opinions and use shame as a disciplinary strategy (Leung *et al.*, 1994), but this association was not found for Chinese/Chinese-American children. In China, research has indicated that shy-inhibited children are more accepted than their peers and more likely to be considered for leadership and considered competent, in contrast to the findings in Western countries. Purely demographic variables may also play a role.

Problems in developing social skills, or 'social fluency', may be a cause of some social anxiety disorder, through either inability or lack of confidence to interact socially and gain positive reactions and acceptance from others. The studies have been mixed, however, with some studies not finding significant problems in social skills while others have. What does seem clear is that the socially anxious perceive their own social skills to be low. It may be that the increasing need for sophisticated social skills in forming relationships or careers, and an emphasis on assertiveness and competitiveness, is making social anxiety problems more common, at least among the 'middle classes'. An interpersonal or media emphasis on 'normal' or 'attractive' personal characteristics has also been argued to fuel perfectionism and feelings of inferiority or insecurity regarding negative evaluation from others. The need for social acceptance or social standing has been elaborated in other lines of research relating to social anxiety.

Substance Induced

While alcohol initially relieves social phobia, excessive alcohol misuse can worsen social phobia symptoms and can cause panic disorder to develop or worsen during alcohol intoxication and especially during alcohol withdrawal syndrome. This effect is not unique to alcohol but can also occur with long-term use of drugs which have a similar mechanism of action to alcohol such as the benzodiazepines which are sometimes prescribed as tranquillisers. Benzodiazepines possess anti-anxiety properties and can be useful for the short-term treatment of severe anxiety. Like the anticonvulsants, they tend to be mild and well tolerated, although there is a risk of habit-forming. Benzodiazepines are usually administered orally for the treatment of anxiety; however, occasionally lorazepam or diazepam may be given intravenously for the treatment of panic attacks.

The World Council of Anxiety does not recommend benzodiazepines for the long-term treatment of anxiety due to a range of problems associated with long-term use including tolerance, psychomotor impairment, cognitive and memory impairments, physical dependence and a benzodiazepine withdrawal syndrome upon discontinuation of benzodiazepines. Despite increasing focus on the use of antidepressants and other agents for the treatment of anxiety, benzodiazepines have remained a mainstay of anxiolytic pharmacotherapy due to their robust efficacy, rapid onset of therapeutic effect, and generally favorable side effect profile. Treatment patterns for psychotropic drugs appear to have remained stable over the past decade, with benzodiazepines being the most commonly used medication for panic disorder.

Approximately half of patients attending mental health services for conditions including anxiety disorders such as panic disorder or social phobia are the result of alcohol or benzodiazepine dependence. Sometimes anxiety pre-existed alcohol or benzodiazepine dependence but the alcohol or benzodiazepine dependence act to keep the anxiety disorders going and often progressively making them worse. Many people who are addicted to alcohol or prescribed benzodiazepines when it is explained to them they have a choice between ongoing ill mental health or quitting and recovering from their symptoms decide on quitting alcohol or their benzodiazepines. It was noted that every individual has an individual sensitivity level to alcohol or sedative hypnotic drugs and what one person can tolerate without ill health another will suffer very ill health and that even moderate drinking can cause rebound anxiety syndromes and sleep disorders. A person who is suffering the toxic effects of alcohol or benzodiazepines will not benefit from other therapies or medications as they do not address the root cause of the symptoms. Symptoms may temporarily worsen however, during alcohol withdrawal or benzodiazepine withdrawal.

Psychological Factors

Research has indicated the role of 'core' or 'unconditional' negative beliefs (e.g. "I am inept") and 'conditional' beliefs nearer to the surface (e.g. "If I show myself, I will be rejected"). They are thought to develop based on personality and adverse experiences and to be activated when the person feels under threat. One line of work has focused more specifically on the key role of self-presentational concerns. The resulting anxiety states are seen as interfering with social performance and the ability to concentrate on interaction, which in turn creates more social problems, which strengthens the negative schema. Also highlighted has been a high focus on and worry about anxiety symptoms themselves and how they might appear to others. A similar model emphasizes the development of a distorted mental representation of the self and overestimates of the likelihood and consequences of negative evaluation, and of the performance standards that others have. Such cognitive-behavioral models consider the role of negatively biased memories of the past and the processes of rumination after an event, and fearful anticipation before it. Studies have also highlighted the role of subtle avoidance and defensive factors, and shown how attempts to avoid feared negative evaluations or use of 'safety behaviors' (Clark & Wells, 1995) can make social interaction more difficult and the anxiety worse in the long run. This work has been influential in the development of Cognitive Behavioral Therapy for social anxiety disorder, which has been shown to have efficacy.

Mechanisms

There are many studies investigating neural bases of social anxiety disorder. Although the exact neural mechanisms have not been found yet, there is evidence relating social anxiety disorder to imbalance in some neurochemicals and hyperactivity in some brain areas.

Neurotransmitters

Sociability is closely tied to dopamine neurotransmission. Misuse of stimulants like amphetamines to increase self-confidence and improve social performance is common. In a recent study a direct relation between social status of volunteers and binding affinity of dopamine D2/3 receptors in the striatum was found. Other research shows that the binding affinity of dopamine D2 receptors in the striatum of social anxiety sufferers is lower than in controls. Some other research shows an abnormality in dopamine transporter density in the striatum of social anxiety sufferers. However, some researchers have been unable to replicate previous findings of evidence of dopamine abnormality in social anxiety disorder. Studies have shown high prevalence of social anxiety in Parkinson's disease and schizophrenia. In a recent study, social phobia was diagnosed in 50% of Parkinson's disease patients. Other researchers have found social phobia symptoms in patients treated with dopamine antagonists like haloperidol, emphasizing the role of dopamine neurotransmission in social anxiety disorder. Also, concentration problems, mental and physical fatigue, anhedonia and decreased self-confidence can be seen in those with social anxiety disorder.

Some evidence points to the possibility that social anxiety disorder involves reduced serotonin receptor binding. A recent study reports increased serotonin transporter binding in psychotropic medication-naive patients with generalized social anxiety disorder. Although there is little evidence of abnormality in serotonin neurotransmission, the limited efficacy of medications which affect serotonin levels may indicate the role of this pathway. Paroxetine and sertraline are two SSRIs that have been confirmed by the FDA to treat social anxiety disorder. Some researchers believe that SSRIs decrease the activity of the amygdala.

There is also increasing focus on other candidate transmitters, e.g. norepinephrine and glutamate, which may be over-active in social anxiety disorder, and the inhibitory transmitter GABA, which may be under-active in the thalamus.

Brain Areas

The amygdala is part of the limbic system which is related to fear cognition and emotional learning. Individuals with social anxiety disorder have been found to have a hypersensitive amygdala; for example in relation to social threat cues (e.g. perceived negative evaluation by another person), angry or hostile faces, and while waiting to give a speech. Recent research has also indicated that another area of the brain, the anterior cingulate cortex, which was already known to be involved in the experience of physical pain, also appears to be involved in the experience of 'social pain', for example perceiving group exclusion. A 2007 meta-analysis also found that individuals with social anxiety had hyperactiviation in the amygdala and insula areas which are frequently associated with fear and negative emotional processing.

Diagnosis

ICD-10 defines social phobia as a fear of scrutiny by other people leading to avoidance of social situations. The anxiety symptoms may present as a complaint of blushing, hand tremor, nausea or urgency of micturition. Symptoms may progress to panic attacks.

Standardized rating scales such as the Social Phobia Inventory, the SPAI-B, Liebowitz Social Anxiety Scale, and the Social Interaction Anxiety Scale can be used to screen for social anxiety disorder and measure the severity of anxiety.

Prevention

Prevention of anxiety disorders is one focus of research. Use of CBT and related techniques may decrease the number of children with social anxiety disorder following completion of prevention programs.

Treatment

Psychotherapies

The first line treatment for social anxiety disorder is cognitive behavioral therapy with medications such as selective serotonin reuptake inhibitors (SSRIs) used only in those who are not interested in therapy. Self-help based on principles of CBT is a second-line treatment.

There is some emerging evidence for the use of Acceptance and Commitment Therapy (ACT) in the treatment of social anxiety disorder. ACT Is considered an offshoot of traditional CBT and emphasizes accepting unpleasant symptoms rather than fighting against them, as well as psychological flexibility - the ability to adapt to changing situational demands, to shift one's perspective, and to balance competing desires. ACT may be useful as a second line treatment for this disorder in situations where CBT is ineffective or refused.

Some studies have suggested social skills training (SST) can help with social anxiety. Examples of social skills focused on during SST for social anxiety disorder include: initiating conversations, establishing friendships, interacting with members of the opposite sex, constructing a speech and assertiveness skills. However, it is not clear whether specific social skills techniques and training are required, rather than just support with general social functioning and exposure to social situations.

Given the evidence that social anxiety disorder may predict subsequent development of other psychiatric disorders such as depression, early diagnosis and treatment is important. Social anxiety disorder remains under-recognized in primary care practice, with patients often presenting for treatment only after the onset of complications such as clinical depression or substance abuse disorders.

A 2014 systematic review of interventions for adults with social anxiety disorder identified following psychotherapic interventions from published and unpublished sources. Outcomes were validated measures of social anxiety, reported as standardised mean differences compared with waitlist.

Intervention	Trials	Participants	Effect
Exercise promotion	1	18	-0.36
Exposure and social skills	10	227	-0.86
Exposure in vivo	9	199	-0.83
Social skills training	1	28	-0.88
Group cognitive behavioural therapy	28	984	-0.92
Heimberg model	11	338	-0.80
Other (no model specified)	16	583	-0.85
Enhanced cognitive behavioral therapy	1	63	-1.10
Individual cognitive behavioral therapy	15	562	-1.19
Hope, Heimberg and Turk Model	2	53	-1.02
Other (no model specified)	6	163	-1.19
Clark and Wells cognitive therapy model	3	97	-1.56
Clark and Wells cognitive therapy shortened sessions	4	249	-0.97
Other psychological therapy	7	182	-0.36
Interpersonal psychotherapy	2	64	-0.43
Mindfulness training	3	64	-0.39
Supportive therapy	2	54	-0.26
Psychodynamic psychotherapy	3	185	-0.62
Self-help with support	16	748	-0.86
Book with support	3	52	-0.85

Internet with support	13	696	-0.88
Self-help without support	9	406	-0.75
Book without support	4	136	-0.84
Internet without support	5	270	-0.66

Medications

SSRIs

Selective serotonin reuptake inhibitors (SSRIs), a class of antidepressants, are first choice medication for generalized social phobia but a second line treatment. Compared to older forms of medication, there is less risk of tolerability and drug dependency associated with SSRIs.

In a 1995 double-blind, placebo-controlled trial, the SSRI paroxetine was shown to result in clinically meaningful improvement in 55 percent of patients with generalized social anxiety disorder, compared with 23.9 percent of those taking placebo. An October 2004 study yielded similar results. Patients were treated with either fluoxetine, psychotherapy, or a placebo. The first four sets saw improvement in 50.8 to 54.2 percent of the patients. Of those assigned to receive only a placebo, 31.7 percent achieved a rating of 1 or 2 on the Clinical Global Impression-Improvement scale. Those who sought both therapy and medication did not see a boost in improvement.

General side-effects are common during the first weeks while the body adjusts to the drug. Symptoms may include headaches, nausea, insomnia and changes in sexual behavior. Treatment safety during pregnancy has not been established. In late 2004 much media attention was given to a proposed link between SSRI use and suicidality [a term that encompasses suicidal ideation and attempts at suicide as well as suicide]. For this reason, [although evidential causality between SSRI use and actual suicide has not been demonstrated] the use of SSRIs in pediatric cases of depression is now recognized by the Food and Drug Administration as warranting a cautionary statement to the parents of children who may be prescribed SSRIs by a family doctor. Recent studies have shown no increase in rates of suicide. These tests, however, represent those diagnosed with depression, not necessarily with social anxiety disorder.

In addition, studies show that more socially phobic patients treated with anti-depressant medication develop hypomania than non-phobic controls. The hypomania can be seen as the medication creating a new problem.

Other Drugs

Other prescription drugs are also used, if other methods are not effective. Before the introduction of SSRIs, monoamine oxidase inhibitors (MAOIs) such as phenelzine were frequently used in the treatment of social anxiety. Evidence continues to indicate that MAOIs are effective in the treatment and management of social anxiety disorder and they are still used, but generally only as a last resort medication, owing to concerns about dietary restrictions, possible adverse drug interactions and because of the need for multiple doses per day. A newer type of this medication, Reversible inhibitors of monoamine oxidase subtype A (RIMAs) such as the drug moclobemide, bind reversibly to the MAO-A enzyme, greatly reducing the risk of hypertensive crisis with dietary tyramine intake.

Benzodiazepines such as clonazepam are an alternative to SSRIs. These drugs are often used for short-term relief of severe, disabling anxiety. Although benzodiazepines are still sometimes prescribed for long-term everyday use in some countries, there is concern over the development of drug tolerance, dependency and misuse. It has been recommended that benzodiazepines be considered only for individuals who fail to respond to other medications. Benzodiazepines augment the action of GABA, the major inhibitory neurotransmitter in the brain; effects usually begin to appear within minutes or hours. In most patients, tolerance rapidly develops to the sedative effects of benzodiazepines, but not to the anxiolytic effects. Long-term use of benzodiazepine may result in physical dependence, and abrupt discontinuation of the drug should be avoided due to high potential for withdrawal symptoms (including tremor, insomnia, and in rare cases, seizures). A gradual tapering of the dose of clonazepam (a decrease of 0.25 mg every 2 weeks), however, has been shown to be well tolerated by patients with social anxiety disorder. Benzodiazepines are not recommended as monotherapy for patients who have major depression in addition to social anxiety disorder and should be avoided in patients with a history of substance abuse.

Certain anticonvulsant drugs such as gabapentin are effective in social anxiety disorder and may be a possible treatment alternative to benzodiazepines.

Serotonin-norepinephrine reuptake inhibitors (SNRIs) such as venlafaxine have shown similar effectiveness to the SSRIs. In Japan, Milnacipran is used in the treatment of Taijin kyofusho, a Japanese variant of social anxiety disorder. The atypical antidepressants mirtazapine and bupropion have been studied for the treatment of social anxiety disorder, and rendered mixed results.

Some people with a form of social phobia called performance phobia have been helped by beta-blockers, which are more commonly used to control high blood pressure. Taken in low doses, they control the physical manifestation of anxiety and can be taken before a public performance.

A novel treatment approach has recently been developed as a result of translational research. It has been shown that a combination of acute dosing of d-cycloserine (DCS) with exposure therapy facilitates the effects of exposure therapy of social phobia. DCS is an old antibiotic medication used for treating tuberculosis and does not have any anxiolytic properties per se. However, it acts as an agonist at the glutamatergic N-methyl-D-aspartate (NMDA) receptor site, which is important for learning and memory.

Kava-kava has also attracted attention as a possible treatment, although safety concerns exist.

Epidemiology

Country	Prevalence
United States	2–7%
England	0.4% (children)
Scotland	1.8% (children)
Wales	0.6% (children)
Australia	1–2.7%
Brazil	4.7–7.9%
India	12.8% (adolescents)
Iran	0.8%
Israel	4.5%
Nigeria	9.4% (university students)
Sweden	15.6%
Turkey	9.6% (university students)
Poland	7-9% (2002)
Taiwan	7% children (2002~2008)

Social anxiety disorder is known to appear at an early age in most cases. Fifty percent of those who develop this disorder have developed it by the age of 11, and 80% have developed it by age 20. This early age of onset may lead to people with social anxiety disorder being particularly vulnerable to depressive illnesses, drug abuse and other psychological conflicts.

When prevalence estimates were based on the examination of psychiatric clinic samples, social anxiety disorder was thought to be a relatively rare disorder. The opposite was found to be true; social anxiety was common, but many were afraid to seek psychiatric help, leading to an underrecognition of the problem.

The National Comorbidity Survey of over 8,000 American correspondents in 1994 revealed 12-month and lifetime prevalence rates of 7.9 percent and 13.3 percent, respectively; this makes it the third most prevalent psychiatric disorder after depression and alcohol dependence, and the most common of the anxiety disorders. According to U.S. epidemiological data from the National Institute of Mental Health, social phobia affects 15 million adult Americans in any given year. Estimates vary within 2 percent and 7 percent of the U.S. adult population.

The mean onset of social phobia is 10 to 13 years. Onset after age 25 is rare and is typically preceded by panic disorder or major depression. Social anxiety disorder occurs more often in females than males. The prevalence of social phobia appears to be increasing among white, married, and well-educated individuals. As a group, those with generalized social phobia are less likely to graduate from high school and are more likely to rely on government financial assistance or have poverty-level salaries. Surveys carried out in 2002 show the youth of England, Scotland, and Wales have a prevalence rate of 0.4 percent, 1.8 percent, and 0.6 percent, respectively. In Canada, the prevalence of self-reported social anxiety for Nova Scotians older than 14 years was 4.2 percent in June 2004 with women (4.6 percent) reporting more than men (3.8 percent). In Australia, social phobia is the 8th and 5th leading disease or illness for males and females between 15–24 years of age as of 2003. Because of the difficulty in separating social phobia from poor social skills or shyness, some studies have a large range of prevalence. The table also shows higher prevalence in Brazil.

History

Literary descriptions of shyness can be traced back to the days of Hippocrates around 400 B.C. Hippocrates described someone who "through bashfulness, suspicion, and timorousness, will not be seen abroad; loves darkness as life and cannot endure the light or to sit in lightsome places; his hat still in his eyes, he will neither see, nor be seen by his good will. He dare not come in company for fear he should be misused, disgraced, overshoot himself in gesture or speeches, or be sick; he thinks every man observes him."

The first mention of the psychiatric term social phobia (*phobie des situations sociales*), was made in the early 1900s. Psychologists used the term "social neurosis" to describe extremely shy patients in the 1930s. After extensive work by Joseph Wolpe on systematic desensitization, research on phobias and their treatment grew. The idea that social phobia was a separate entity from other phobias came from the British psychiatrist Isaac Marks, in the 1960s. This was accepted by the American Psychiatric Association and was first officially included in the third edition of the Diagnostic and Statistical Manual of Mental Disorders. The definition of the phobia was revised in 1989 to allow comorbidity with avoidant personality disorder, and introduced generalized social phobia. Social phobia had been largely ignored prior to 1985.

After a call to action by psychiatrist Michael Liebowitz and clinical psychologist Richard Heimberg, there was an increase in attention to and research on the disorder. The DSM-IV gave social phobia the alternative name social anxiety disorder. Research on the psychology and sociology of everyday social anxiety continued. Cognitive Behavioural models and therapies were developed for social anxiety disorder. In the 1990s, paroxetine became the first prescription drug in the U.S. approved to treat social anxiety disorder, with others following.

Separation Anxiety Disorder

Separation anxiety disorder (SAD), is an anxiety disorder in which an individual experiences excessive anxiety regarding separation from home or from people to whom the individual has a strong emotional attachment (e.g. a parent, caregiver, significant other or siblings). It is most common in infants and small children, typically between the ages of 6–7 months to 3 years, although it may pathologically manifest itself in older children, adolescents and adults. Separation anxiety is a natural part of the developmental process. Unlike SAD (indicated by excessive anxiety), normal separation anxiety indicates healthy advancements in a child's cognitive maturation and should not be considered a developing behavioral problem.

According to the American Psychology Association, separation anxiety disorder is an excessive display of fear and distress when faced with situations of separation from the home or from a specific attachment figure. The anxiety that is expressed is categorized as being atypical of the expected developmental level and age. The severity of the symptoms ranges from anticipatory uneasiness to full-blown anxiety about separation.

SAD may cause significant negative effects within areas of social and emotional functioning, family life, and physical health of the disordered individual. The duration of this problem must persist for at least four weeks and must present itself before a child is 18 years of age to be diagnosed as SAD in children, but can now be diagnosed in adults with a duration typically lasting 6 months in adults as specified by the DSM-5.

Signs and Symptoms

Academic Setting

As with other anxiety disorders, children with SAD face more obstacles at school than those without anxiety disorders. Adjustment and relating school functioning have been found to be much more difficult for anxious children. In some severe forms of SAD, children may act disruptively in class or may refuse to attend school altogether. It is estimated that nearly 75% of children with SAD exhibit some form of school refusal behavior.

This is a serious problem because, as children fall further behind in coursework, it becomes increasingly difficult for them to return to school.

Short-term problems resulting from academic refusal include poor academic performance or decline in performance, alienation from peers, and conflict within the family.

Although school refusal behavior is common among children with SAD, it is important to note that school refusal behavior is sometimes linked to generalized anxiety disorder or possibly a mood disorder. That being said, a majority of children with separation anxiety disorder have school refusal as a symptom. Up to 80% of children who refuse school qualify for a diagnosis of separation anxiety disorder.

Workplace

Just how SAD affects a child's attendance and participation in school, their avoidance behaviors stay with them as they grow and enter adulthood. Recently, "the effects of mental illness on workplace productivity have become a prominent concern on both the national and international fronts". In general, mental illness is a common health problem among working adults, 20 to 30% of adults will suffer from at least one psychiatric disorder. Mental illness is linked to decreased productivity, and with individuals diagnosed with SAD their levels at which they function decreases dramatically resulting in partial work-days, increase in number of total absences, and "holding back" when it comes to carrying out and completing tasks.

Cause

Factors that contribute to the disorder include a combination and interaction of biological, cognitive, environmental, child temperament, and behavioral factors.

Children are more likely to develop SAD if one or both of their parents was diagnosed with a psychological disorder. Recent research by Daniel Schechter and colleagues have pointed to difficulties of mothers who have themselves had early adverse experiences such as maltreatment and disturbed attachments with their own caregivers, who then go on to develop responses to their infants' and toddlers' normative social bids in the service of social referencing, emotion regulation, and joint attention, which responses are linked to these mothers own psychopathology (i.e. maternal post-traumatic stress disorder (PTSD) and depression. These atypical maternal responses which have been shown to be associated with separation anxiety have been related to disturbances in maternal stress physiologic response to mother-toddler separation as well as lower maternal neural activity in the brain region of the medial prefrontal cortex when mothers with and without PTSD were shown video excerpts of their own and unfamiliar toddlers during mother-child separation versus free-play.

Many psychological professionals have suggested that early and/or traumatic separation from a central caregiver in a child's life can increase the likelihood of them being diagnosed with SAD, school phobia, and depressive-spectrum disorders. Some children can be more vulnerable to SAD due to their temperament, for example, their level of anxiety when placed in new situations.

Environmental

Most often, the onset of separation anxiety disorder is caused by a stressful life-event, especially a loss of a loved one or pet, but can also include parental divorce, change of school or neighborhood, natural disasters, circumstances which forced the individual to be separated from their attachment figure(s). In older individuals, stressful life experiences may include going away to college, moving out for the first time, or becoming a parent.

Genetic and Physiological

There may be a genetic predisposition in children with separation anxiety disorder. "Separation anxiety disorder in children may be heritable." "Heritability was estimated at 73% in a community sample of 6-year-old twins, with higher rates in girls."

A child's temperament can also impact the development of SAD. Timid and shy behaviors may be referred to as "behaviorally inhibited temperaments" in which the child may experience anxiety when they are not familiar with a particular location or person.

Mechanism

Preliminary evidence shows that heightened activity of the amygdala may be associated with symptoms of separation anxiety disorder. Defects in the ventrolateral and dorsomedial areas of the prefrontal cortex are also correlated to anxiety disorders in children.

Diagnosis

Separation anxiety occurs in many infants and young children as they are becoming acclimated with their surroundings. This anxiety is viewed as a normal developmental phase between the months of early infancy until age two. Separation anxiety is normal in young children, until they age 3–4 years, when children are left in a daycare or preschool, away from their parent or primary caregiver. Other sources note that a definite diagnosis of SAD should not be presented until after the age of three. Some studies have shown that hormonal influences during pregnancy can result in lower cortisol levels later in life, which can later lead to psychological disorders, such as SAD. It is also important to note significant life changes experienced by the child either previous to or present at the onset of the disorder. For example, children who emigrated from another country at an early age may have a stronger tendency for developing this disorder, as they have already felt displaced from a location they were starting to become accustomed to. It is not uncommon for them to incessantly cling to their caregiver at first upon arrival to the new location, especially if the child is unfamiliar with the language of their new country. These symptoms may diminish or go away as the child becomes more accustomed to the new surroundings. Other sources note that a definite diagnosis of SAD should not be presented until after the age of three. Separation anxiety may be diagnosed as a disorder if the child's anxiety related to separation from the home or attachment figure is deemed excessive; if the level of anxiety surpasses that of the acceptable caliber for the child's developmental level and age; and if the anxiety negatively impacts the child's everyday life.

Many psychological disorders begin to emerge during childhood. Nearly two-thirds of adults with psychological disorder show signs of their disorder earlier in life. However, not all psychological disorders are present before adulthood. In many cases, there are no signs during childhood.

Behavioral inhibition (BI) plays a large role in many anxiety disorders, SAD included. Compared to children without it, children with BI demonstrate more signs of fear when experiencing a new stimulus, particularly those that are social in nature. Children with BI are at a higher risk for developing a mental disorder, particularly anxiety disorders, than children without BI.

Separation anxiety is normal in young children, until they age 3–4 years, when children are left in a daycare or preschool, away from their parent or primary caregiver.

To be diagnosed with SAD, one must display at least 3 of the following criteria:

- Recurrent excessive distress when anticipating or experiencing separation from home or from major attachment figures

- Persistent and excessive worry about losing major attachment figures or about possible harm to them, such as illness, injury, disasters, or death

- Persistent and excessive worry about experiencing an untoward event (e.g., getting lost, being kidnapped, having an accident, becoming ill) that causes separation from a major attachment figure

- Persistent reluctance or refusal to go out, away from home, to school, to work, or elsewhere because of fear of separation

- Persistent and excessive fear of or reluctance about being alone or without major attachment figures at home or in other settings

- Persistent reluctance or refusal to sleep away from home or to go to sleep without being near a major attachment figure

- Repeated nightmares involving the theme of separation

- Repeated complaints of physical symptoms (e.g., headaches, stomachaches, nausea, vomiting) when separation from major attachment figures occurs or is anticipated

Classification

Separation anxiety is common for infants between the ages of eight and fourteen months and occurs as infants begin to understand their own selfhood—or understand that they are separate persons from their primary caregiver. Infants oftentimes look for their caregivers to give them a sense of comfort and familiarity, which causes separation to become challenging. Subsequently, the concept of object permanence emerges—which is when children learn that something still exists when it cannot be seen or heard, thus increasing their awareness of being separated from their caregiver. Consequently, during the developmental period where an infant's sense self, incorporating object permanence as well, the child also begins to understand that they can in fact be separated from their primary caregiver. They see this separation as something final though, and don't yet understand that their caregiver will return causing fear and distress for the infant. It is when an individual (infant, child, or otherwise) consistently reacts to separation with excessive anxiety and distress and experiences a great deal of interference from their anxiety that a diagnosis of separation anxiety disorder (SAD) can be warranted.

One of the difficulties in the identification of separation anxiety disorder in children is that it highly comorbid with other behavioral disorders, especially generalized anxiety disorder. Behaviors such as refusal or hesitancy in attending school or homesickness for example, can easily reflect similar symptoms and behavioral patterns that are commonly associated with SAD, but could be an overlap of symptoms. The prevalence of co-occurring disorders in adults with separation anxiety disorder is common and includes a much broader spectrum of diagnostic possibilities. Common co-morbidities can include specific phobias, PTSD, panic disorder, obsessive-compulsive disorder, and personality disorders. It is very common for psychological disorders to overlap and even lead to the manifestation of another, especially when it comes to anxiety disorders. Because of the variation and overlap in symptoms a proper, thorough evaluation of the individual is critical to distinguish the differences and significance. An important signifier to establish a difference between SAD and other anxiety or psychological disorders is to investigate where the individual's fear of separation is stemming from; this can be accomplished by asking "what they fear will occur during a separation from their significant other".

What stands out about SAD, as mentioned above, are the avoidance behaviors which present within an individual. Individuals "typically exhibit excessive distress manifested by crying, repeated complaints of physical symptoms (e.g., stomach aches, headaches, etc.), avoidance (e.g., refusing to go to school, to sleep alone, to be left alone in the home, to engage in social events, to go to work, etc.), and engagement in safety behaviors (e.g., frequent calls to or from significant others, and/or primary caregivers)".

Assessment Methods

Assessment methods include diagnostic interviews, self-report measures from both the parent and child, observation of parent-child interaction, and specialized assessment for preschool-aged children. Various facets of a child's development including social life, feeding and sleep schedules, medical issues, traumatic events experienced, family history of mental or anxiety health issues are explored. The compilation of aspects of a child's life aids in capturing a multi-dimensional view of the child's life.

Additionally, while much research has been done in efforts to further understand separation anxiety in regards to the relationship between infants' and their caregivers, it was behavioral psychologist, Mary Ainsworth, who devised a behavioral evaluation method, The Strange Situation (1969), which, at the time, was considered to be the most valuable and famous body of research in the study of separation anxiety. The Strange Situation process assisted in evaluating and measuring the individual attachment styles of infants between the ages of 9 and 18 months. In this observational study, which can be watched by clicking the link ("The Strange Situation Study") below, an environment is created that fluctuates between familiar and unfamiliar situations that would be experienced in everyday life. The variations in stressfulness and the child's responses are observed and, based on the interaction behavior that is directed towards the caregiver, the infant is categorized into one of four different types of attachment styles: 1. Secure (B) 2. Anxious-avoidant, Insecure (A) 3. Anxious-ambivalent/resistant, insecure (C) 4. Disorganized/disoriented (D).

Clinicians may utilize interviews as an assessment tool to gauge the symptomatic occurrences to aid in diagnosing SAD. Interviews may be conducted with the child and also with the attachment figure. Interviewing both child and parent separately allows for the clinician to compile different points of view and information.

Commonly used interviews include:

- Anxiety Disorders Interview Schedule for the DSM-IV, Child Parent Versions (ADIS-IV-C/P)

- Diagnostic Interview Schedule for Children, Version IV (DISC-IV)

- Schedule for Affective Disorders and Schizophrenia for School-aged Children-Present and lifetime version IV (K-SADS-IV)

Self-report Measures

This form of assessment should not be the sole basis of a SAD diagnosis. It is also important to verify that the child who is reporting on their experiences has the cognitive and communication skills appropriate to accurately comprehend and respond to these measurements. An example of a self-report tool that has been tested is: The Separation Anxiety Assessment Scale for Children (SAAS-C). The scale contains 34 items and is divided into six dimensions. The dimensions in order are: Abandonment, Fear of Being Alone, Fear of Physical Illness, Worry about Calamitous Events, Frequency of Calamitous Events, and Safety Signal Index. The first five dimensions have a total of five items while the last one contains nine items. The scale goes beyond assessing symptoms; it focuses on individual cases and treatment planning.

Observation

As noted by Altman, McGoey & Sommer, it is important to observe the child, "in multiple contexts, on numerous occasions, and in their everyday environments (home, daycare, preschool)". It is beneficial to view parent and child interactions and behaviors that may contribute to SAD.

Dyadic Parent-Child Interaction Coding System and recently the Dyadic Parent-Child Interaction Coding System II (DPICS II) are methods used when observing parents and children interactions.

Separation Anxiety Daily Diaries (SADD) have also been used to "assess anxious behaviors along with their antecedents and consequences and may be particularly suited to SAD given its specific focus on parent–child separation" (Silverman & Ollendick, 2005). The diaries are carefully evaluated for validity.

Preschool-aged Children

At the preschool-aged stage, early identification and intervention is crucial. The communication abilities of young children are taken into consideration when creating age-appropriate assessments.

A commonly used assessment tool for preschool-aged children (ages 2–5) is the Preschool Age Psychiatric Assessment (PAPA). Additional questionnaires and rating scales that are used to assess the younger population include the Achenbach Scales, the Fear Survey Schedule for Infants and Preschoolers, and The Infant–Preschool Scale for Inhibited Behaviors.

Preschool children are also interviewed. Two interviews that are sometimes conducted are Attachment Doll-Play and Emotional Knowledge. In both of the assessments the interviewer depicts a scenario where separation and reunion occur; the child is then told to point at one of the four facial expressions presented. These facial expressions show emotions such as anger or sadness. The results are then analyzed.

Behavioral observations are also utilized when assessing the younger population. Observations enable the clinician to view some of the behaviors and emotions in specific contexts.

Treatment

Non-medication based

Non-medication based treatments are the first choice when treating individuals diagnosed with separation anxiety disorder. Counseling tends to be the best replacement for drug treatments. There are two different non-medication approaches to treat separation anxiety. The first is a psychoeducational intervention, often used in conjunction with other therapeutic treatments. This specifically involves educating the individual and their family so that they are knowledgeable about the disorder, as well as parent counseling and guiding teachers on how to help the child. The second is a psychotherapeutic intervention when prior attempts are not effective. Psychotherapeutic interventions are more structured and include behavioral, cognitive-behavioral, contingency, psychodynamic psychotherapy, and family therapy.

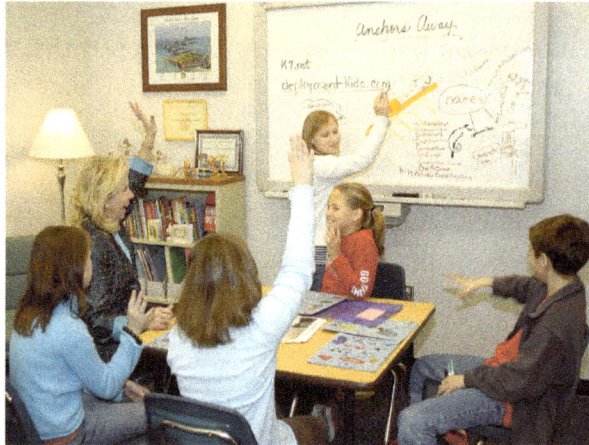

Anchors Away program for children with anxiety disorder.

Behavioral Therapy

Behavioral therapies are types of non-medication based treatment which are mainly exposure-based techniques. These include techniques such as systematic desensitization, emotive imagery, participant modelling and contingency management. Behavioral therapies carefully expose individuals by small increments to slowly reduce their anxiety over time and mainly focuses on their behavior.

Contingency Management

Contingency management is a form of treatment found to be effective for younger children with SAD. Contingency management revolves around a reward system with verbal or tangible reinforcement requiring parental involvement. A contingency contract is written up between the parent and the child, which entails a written agreement about specific goals that the child will try to achieve and the specific reward the parent will provide once the task is accomplished. When the child undergoing contingency management show signs of independence or achieve their treatment goals, they are praised or given their reward. This facilitates a new positive experience with what used to be filled with fear and anxiety. Children in preschool who show symptoms of SAD do not have the communicative ability to express their emotions or the self-control ability to cope with their separation anxiety on their own, so parental involvement is crucial in younger cases of SAD.

Cognitive Behavioral Therapy

Cognitive behavioral therapy (CBT) focuses on helping children with SAD reduce feelings of anxiety through practices of exposure to anxiety-inducing situations and active metacognition to reduce anxious thoughts.

CBT has 3 phases: education, application and relapse prevention. In the education phase, the individual is informed on the different effects anxiety can have physically and more importantly mentally. By understanding and being able to recognize their reactions, it will help to manage and eventually reduce their overall response.

According to Kendall and colleagues, there are four components which must be taught to a child undergoing CBT:

1. Recognizing anxious feelings and behaviors

2. Discussing situations that provoke anxious behaviors

3. Developing a coping plan with appropriate reactions to situations

4. Evaluating effectiveness of the coping plan

In the application phase, individuals can take what they know and apply it in real time situations for helpful exposure. The most important aspect of this phase is for the individuals to ultimately manage themselves throughout the process. In the relapse prevention phase, the individual is informed that continued exposure and application of what worked for them is the key to continual progress.

A study investigated the content of thoughts in anxious children who suffered from separation anxiety as well as from social phobia and/or generalized anxiety. The results suggested that cognitive therapy for children suffering from separation anxiety (along with social phobia and generalized anxiety) should be aimed at identifying negative cognition of one's own behavior in the threat of anxiety-evoking situations and to modify these thoughts to promote self-esteem and ability to properly cope with the given situation.

Cognitive procedures are a form of treatment found to be ideal for older children with SAD. The theory behind this technique is that the child's dysfunctional thoughts, attitudes, and beliefs are what lead to anxiety and cause anxious behavior. Children who are being treated with cognitive procedures are taught to ask themselves if there is "evidence" to support their anxious thoughts and behaviors. They are taught "coping thoughts" to replace previously distorted thoughts during anxiety-inducing situations such as doing a reality check to assess the realistic danger of a situation and then to praise themselves for handling the situation bravely. Examples of such disordered thoughts include polarized thinking, overgeneralization, filtering (focusing on negative), jumping to conclusions, catastrophizing, emotional reasoning, labeling, "shoulds", and placing blame on self and others. Sometimes therapists will involve parents and teach them behavioral tactics such as contingency management.

Medication

The use of medication is applied in extreme cases of SAD when other treatment options have been utilized and failed. However, it has been difficult to prove the benefits of drug treatment in patients with SAD because there have been many mixed results. Despite all the studies and testings, there has yet to be a specific medication for SAD. Medication prescribed for adults from the Food and Drug Administration (FDA) are often used and have been reported to show positive results for children and adolescents with SAD.

There are mixed results regarding the benefits of using tricyclic antidepressants (TCAs), which includes imipramine and clomipramine. One study suggested that imipramine is helpful for children with "school phobia," who also had an underlying diagnosis of SAD. However, other studies have also shown that imipramine and clonipramine had the same effect of children who were treated with the medication and placebo. The most promising medication is the use of selective serotonin reuptake inhibitors (SSRI) in adults and children. Several studies have shown that patients treated with fluvoxamine were significantly better than those treated with placebo. They showed decreasing anxiety symptoms with short-term and long-term use of the medication.

Prognosis

Discomfort from separations in children from ages 8 to 14 months is normal. Children oftentimes get nervous or afraid of unfamiliar people and places but if the behavior still occurs after the age of 6 and if it lasts longer than four weeks, the child might have Separation Anxiety Disorder. About 4% of children have the disorder. Separation Anxiety Disorder is very treatable especially when caught early on with medication and behavioral therapies. Helping children with separation anxiety to identify the circumstances that elicit their anxiety (upcoming separation events) is important. A child's ability to tolerate separations should gradually increase over time when he or she is gradually exposed to the feared events. Encouraging a child with separation anxiety disorder to feel competent and empowered, as well as to discuss feelings associated with anxiety-provoking events promotes recovery.

Children with separation anxiety disorder often respond negatively to perceived anxiety in their caretakers, in that parents and caregivers who also have anxiety disorders may unwittingly confirm a child's unrealistic fears that something terrible may happen if they are separated from each other. Thus, it is critical that parents and caretakers become aware of their own feelings and communicate a sense of safety and confidence about separation.

Longitudinal effects

Several studies aim to understand the long-term mental health consequences of SAD. SAD contributed to vulnerability and acted as a strong risk factor for developing other mental disorders in people aged 19–30. Specifically disorders including panic disorder and depressive disorders were more likely to occur. Other sources also support the increased likelihood of displaying either of the two psychopathologies with previous history of childhood SAD.

Epidemiology

Anxiety disorders are the most common type of psychopathology to occur in today's youth, affecting from 5–25% of children worldwide. Of these anxiety disorders, SAD accounts for a large proportion of diagnoses. SAD may account for up to 50% of the anxiety disorders as recorded in referrals for mental health treatment. SAD is noted as one of the earliest-occurring of all anxiety disorders. Adult separation anxiety disorder affects roughly 7% of adults. It has also been reported that the clinically anxious pediatric population are considerably larger. For example, according to Hammerness et al. (2008) SAD accounted for 49% of admissions.

Research suggests that 4.1% of children will experience a clinical level of separation anxiety. Of that 4.1% it is calculated that nearly a third of all cases will persist into adulthood if left untreated. Research continues to explore the implications that early dispositions of SAD in childhood may serve as risk factors for the development of mental disorders throughout adolescence and adulthood. It is presumed that a much higher percentage of children suffer from a small amount of separation anxiety, and are not actually diagnosed. Multiple studies have found higher rates of SAD in girls than in boys, and that paternal absence may increase the chances of SAD in girls.

Generalized Anxiety Disorder

Generalized anxiety disorder (GAD) is an anxiety disorder characterized by excessive, uncontrollable and often irrational worry, that is, apprehensive expectation about events or activities. This excessive worry often interferes with daily functioning, as individuals with GAD typically anticipate disaster, and are overly concerned about everyday matters such as health issues, money, death, family problems, friendship problems, interpersonal relationship problems, or work difficulties. Individuals often exhibit a variety of physical symptoms, including fatigue, fidgeting, headaches, nausea, numbness in hands and feet, muscle tension, muscle aches, difficulty swallowing, excessive stomach acid buildup, stomach pain, vomiting, diarrhea, bouts of breathing difficulty, difficulty concentrating, trembling, twitching, irritability, agitation, sweating, restlessness, insomnia, hot flashes, rashes, and inability to fully control the anxiety (ICD-10). These symptoms must be consistent and ongoing, persisting at least six months, for a formal diagnosis of GAD.

Standardized rating scales such as GAD-7 can be used to assess severity of GAD symptoms. GAD is the most common cause of disability in the workplace in the United States.

In a given year, approximately two percent of American adults and European adults experience GAD. Globally about 4% are affected at some point in their life. GAD is seen in women twice as much as men. GAD is also common in individuals with a history of substance abuse and a family history of the disorder. Once GAD develops, it may become chronic, but can be managed or eliminated with proper treatment.

Causes

Genetics

About a third of the variance for generalized anxiety disorder has been attributed to genes. Individuals with a genetic predisposition for GAD are more likely to develop GAD, especially in response to a life stressor.

Substance-induced

Long-term use of benzodiazepines can worsen underlying anxiety, with evidence that reduction of benzodiazepines can lead to a lessening of anxiety symptoms. Similarly, long-term alcohol use is associated with anxiety disorders, with evidence that prolonged abstinence can result in a disappearance of anxiety symptoms. However, it can take up to two years for anxiety symptoms to return to baseline in about a quarter of people recovering from alcoholism.

In one study in 1988–90, illness in approximately half of patients attending mental health services at British hospital psychiatric clinic, for conditions including anxiety disorders such as panic disorder or social phobia, was determined to be the result of alcohol or benzodiazepine dependence. In these patients, anxiety symptoms, while worsening initially during the withdrawal phase, disappeared with abstinence from benzodiazepines or alcohol. Sometimes anxiety pre-existed alcohol or benzodiazepine dependence, but the dependence was acting to keep the anxiety disorders going and often progressively making them worse. Recovery from benzodiazepines tends to take a lot longer than recovery from alcohol, but people can regain their previous good health.

Tobacco smoking has been established as a risk factor for developing anxiety disorders.

Excessive caffeine usage has been linked to anxiety.

Mechanisms

Generalized anxiety disorder has been linked to disrupted functional connectivity of the amygdala and its processing of fear and anxiety. Sensory information enters the amygdala through the nuclei of the basolateral complex (consisting of lateral, basal and accessory basal nuclei). The basolateral complex processes the sensory-related fear memories and communicates their threat importance to memory and sensory processing elsewhere in the brain, such as the medial prefrontal cortex and sensory cortices.

Another area, the adjacent central nucleus of the amygdala, controls species-specific fear responses in its connections to the brainstem, hypothalamus and cerebellum areas. In those with generalized anxiety disorder, these connections seem less functionally distinct, and there is greater gray matter in the central nucleus. Another difference is that the amygdala areas have decreased connectivity with the insula and cingulate areas that control general stimulus salience, while having greater connectivity with the parietal cortex and prefrontal cortex circuits that underlie executive functions. The latter suggests a compensation strategy for dysfunctional amygdala processing of anxiety. This is consistent with cognitive theories that suggest the use in this disorder of attempts to reduce the involvement of emotions with compensatory cognitive strategies.

Diagnosis

DSM-5 Criteria

The diagnostic criteria for GAD as defined by the Diagnostic and Statistical Manual of Mental Disorders DSM-5 (2013), published by the American Psychiatric Association, are paraphrased as follows:

A. Too much anxiety or worry over more than six months. This is present most of the time in regards to many activities.

B. Inability to manage these symptoms

C. At least three of the following occur:

   1. Restlessness

   2. Tires easily

   3. Problems concentrating

   4. Irritability

   5. Muscle tension.

   6. Problems with sleep

D. Symptoms result in problems with functioning.

E. Symptoms are not due to medications, drugs, other physical health problems

F. Symptoms do not fit better with another psychiatric problem such as panic disorder

No major changes to GAD have occurred since publication of the Diagnostic and Statistical Manual of Mental Disorders (2004); minor changes include wording of diagnostic criteria.

ICD-10 Criteria

ICD-10 Generalized anxiety disorder "F41.1"

A. A period of at least six months with prominent tension, worry, and feelings of apprehension, about everyday events and problems.

B. At least four symptoms out of the following list of items must be present, of which at least one from items (1) to (4).

Autonomic arousal symptoms

1. Palpitations or pounding heart, or accelerated heart rate.

2. Sweating.

3. Trembling or shaking.

4. Dry mouth (not due to medication or dehydration).

Symptoms concerning chest and abdomen

5. Difficulty breathing.

6. Feeling of choking.

7. Chest pain or discomfort.

8. Nausea or abdominal distress (e.g. churning in the stomach).

Symptoms concerning brain and mind

9. Feeling dizzy, unsteady, faint or light-headed.

10. Feelings that objects are unreal (derealization), or that one's self is distant or "not really here" (depersonalization).

11. Fear of losing control, going crazy, or passing out.

12. Fear of dying.

General symptoms

13. Hot flashes or cold chills.

14. Numbness or tingling sensations.

Symptoms of tension

15. Muscle tension or aches and pains.

16. Restlessness and inability to relax.

17. Feeling keyed up, or on edge, or of mental tension.

18. A sensation of a lump in the throat or difficulty with swallowing.

Other non-specific symptoms

19. Exaggerated response to minor surprises or being startled.

20. Difficulty in concentrating or mind going blank, because of worrying or anxiety.

21. Persistent irritability.

22. Difficulty getting to sleep because of worrying.

C. The disorder does not meet the criteria for panic disorder (F41.0), phobic anxiety disorders (F40.-), obsessive-compulsive disorder (F42.-) or hypochondriacal disorder (F45.2).

D. Most commonly used exclusion criteria: not sustained by a physical disorder, such as hyperthyroidism, an organic mental disorder (F0) or psychoactive substance-related disorder (F1), such as excess consumption of amphetamine-like substances, or withdrawal from benzodiazepines.

History of Diagnosis

The American Psychiatric Association first introduced GAD as a diagnosis in the DSM-III in 1980. Prior to the introduction of this diagnosis, GAD was presented as one of the two core components of anxiety neurosis, the other being panic. The definition in the DSM-III required uncontrollable and diffuse anxiety or worry that is excessive and unrealistic and persists for 1 month or longer. High rates in comorbidity of GAD and major depression led many commentators to suggest that GAD would be better conceptualized as an aspect of major depression instead of an independent disorder. Many critics stated that the diagnostic features of this disorder were not well established until the DSM-III-R. Since comorbidity of GAD and other disorders decreased with time, the DSM-III-R changed the time requirement for a GAD diagnosis to 6 months or longer.

The DSM-IV changed the definition of *excessive worry* and the number of associated psychophysiological symptoms required for a diagnosis. Another aspect of the diagnosis the DSM-IV clarified was what constitutes a symptom as occurring "often." The DSM-IV also required difficulty controlling the worry to be diagnosed with GAD. The DSM-5 emphasized that excessive worrying had to occur more days than not and on a number of different topics. It has been stated that the constant changes in the diagnostic features of the disorder have made it difficult for researchers to identify the biological and psychological underpinnings of the disorder making it difficult to create specialized medications for the disorder. This has led to the continuation of GAD being medicated heavily with SSRIs.

Prevention

Mental disorders are difficult to prevent, but many techniques are available to help relieve and manage anxiety. Many sufferers have found ease by relaxation exercises, deep breathing practice and meditation. Additionally, avoidance of caffeine may prevent GAD. Avoiding nicotine also can decrease the risk for the development of anxiety disorders including generalized anxiety disorder.

Treatment

Meta-analysis indicates that both cognitive behavioral therapy (CBT) and medications (such as SSRIs) have been shown to be effective in reducing anxiety. A comparison of overall outcomes of CBT and medication on anxiety did not show statistically significant differences (i.e. they were equally effective in treating anxiety). However, CBT is significantly more effective in reducing depression severity, and its effects are more likely to be maintained in the long term, whereas the effectiveness of pharmacologic treatment tends to lessen if medication is discontinued. A combination of both CBT and medication is generally seen as the most desirable approach to treatment. Use of medication to lower extreme anxiety levels can be important in enabling patients to engage effectively in CBT.

Therapy

Generalized anxiety disorder is based on psychological components that include cognitive avoidance, positive worry beliefs, ineffective problem-solving and emotional processing, interpersonal issues, previous trauma, intolerance of uncertainty, negative problem orientation, ineffective coping, emotional hyperarousal, poor understanding of emotions, negative cognitive reactions to emotions, maladaptive emotion management and regulation, experiential avoidance, and behavioral restriction. To combat the previous cognitive and emotional aspects of GAD, psychologists often include some of the following key treatment components in their intervention plan; self-monitoring, relaxation techniques, self-control desensitization, gradual stimulus control, cognitive restructuring, worry outcome monitoring, present-moment focus, expectancy-free living, problem-solving techniques, processing of core fears, social-ization, discussion and reframing of worry beliefs, emotional skills training, experi-ential exposure, psychoeducation, mindfulness and acceptance exercises. There exist behavioral, cognitive, and a combination of both treatments for GAD that focus on some of those key components.

Among the cognitive–behavioral orientated psychotherapies the two main treatments are cognitive behavioral therapy and acceptance and commitment therapy (ACT). In-tolerance of uncertainty therapy and motivational interviewing are two new treatments for GAD that are used as either stand-alone treatments or additional strategies that may enhance CBT.

Cognitive Behavioral Therapy

Cognitive behavioral therapy (CBT) is a psychological method of treatment for GAD that involves a therapist working with the patient to understand how thoughts and feelings influence behaviour. Elements of the therapy include exposure strategies to allow the patient to confront their anxieties gradually and feel more comfortable in anxiety-provoking situations, as well as to practice the skills they have learned. CBT can be used alone or in conjunction with medication.

Components of CBT for GAD includes psychoeducation, self-monitoring, stimulus con-trol techniques, relaxation, self-control desensitization, cognitive restructuring, worry exposure, worry behavior modification, and problem-solving. The first step in the treat-ment of GAD is informing of the patient about the issues and the plan of the solution. The purpose of psychoeducation is to provide some relief, destigmatization of the dis-order, motivating, and accomplishing participation by making the patient understand the program of treatment. The purpose of this component is to identify cues that pro-voke the anxiety. Stimulus control intervention refers to minimizing the stimulus con-ditions under which worrying occurs. Relaxation techniques lower the patients' stress and thus increase attention to alternatives in feared situations (other than worrying). Deep breathing exercise, progressive muscle relaxation, and applied relaxation fall un-der the scope of relaxation techniques.

Self-control desensitization involves patients being deeply relaxed before vividly imagining themselves in situations that usually make them anxious and worry until internal anxiety cues are triggered. Patients then imagine themselves coping with the situation and decreasing their anxious response. If anxiety diminishes, they then enter a deeper relaxed state and turn off the scene. The purpose of cognitive restruc-turing is to shift from a worrisome outlook to a more functional and adaptive per-ception of the world, the future, and the self. It involves Socratic questioning that leads patients to think through their worries and anxieties so they can realize that alternative interpretations and feelings are more accurate. It also involves behav-ioral experiments that actually test the validity of both the negative and alternative thoughts in real-life situations. In CBT for GAD, patients also engage in worry exposure exercises during which they are asked to imagine themselves exposed to images of the most feared outcomes. Then they engage in response-prevention instruction that prevents them from avoiding the image and motivates alternative outcomes to the feared stimulus. The goals of worry exposure are habituation and reinterpretation of the meaning of the feared stimulus. Worry behavior prevention requires patients to monitor the behaviors that caused them worry and are then asked to prevent themselves from engaging in them. Instead, they are encouraged to use other coping mechanisms learned earlier in the treatment. Finally, problem solving focuses on dealing with current problems through a problem-solving approach: (1) definition of the problem, (2) formulation of goals, (3) creation of alternative solutions, (4) decision-making, and (5) implementing and verifying the solutions.

There is little debate regarding the effectiveness of CBT for GAD. However, there is still room for improvement because only about 50% of those who complete treatments achieve higher functioning or recovery after treatment. Therefore, there's a need for enhancement of current components of CBT. CBT usually helps one-third of the patients substantially, whilst another third does not respond at all to treatment.

Acceptance and Commitment Therapy

Acceptance and commitment therapy (ACT) is a behavioral treatment based on acceptance-based models. ACT is designed with the purpose to target three therapeutic goals: (1) reduce the use of avoiding strategies intended to avoid feelings, thoughts, memories, and sensations; (2) decreasing a person's literal response to their thoughts (e.g., understanding that thinking "I'm hopeless" does not mean that the person's life is truly hopeless), and (3) increasing the person's ability to keep commitments to changing their behaviors. These goals are attained by switching the person's attempt to control events to working towards changing their behavior and focusing on valued directions and goals in their lives as well as committing to behaviors that help the individual accomplish those personal goals. This psychological therapy teaches mindfulness (paying attention on purpose, in the present, and in a nonjudgmental manner) and acceptance (openness and willingness to sustain contact) skills for responding to uncontrollable events and therefore manifesting behaviors that enact personal values. Like many other psychological therapies, ACT works best in combination with pharmacology treatments.

Intolerance of Uncertainty Therapy

Intolerance of uncertainty therapy (IUT) refers to a consistent negative reaction to uncertain and ambiguous events regardless of their likelihood of occurrence. IUT is used as a stand-alone treatment for GAD patients. Thus, IUT focuses on helping patients in developing the ability to tolerate, cope with and accept uncertainty in their life in order to reduce anxiety. IUT is based on the psychological components of psychoeducation, awareness of worry, problem-solving training, re-evaluation of the usefulness of worry, imagining virtual exposure, recognition of uncertainty, and behavioral exposure. Studies have shown support for the efficacy of this therapy with GAD patients with continued improvements in follow-up periods.

Motivational Interviewing

A promising innovative approach to improving recovery rates for the treatment of GAD is to combine CBT with motivational interviewing (MI). Motivational interviewing is a strategy centered on the patient that aims to increase intrinsic motivation and decrease ambivalence about change due to the treatment. MI contains four key elements: (1) express empathy, (2) heighten dissonance between behaviors that are not desired and values that are not consistent with those behaviors, (3) move with resistance rather than direct confrontation, and (4) encourage self-efficacy. It is based on asking open-ended questions and listening carefully and reflectively to patients' answers, eliciting "change talk", and talking with patients about the pros and cons of change. Some studies have shown the combination of CBT with MI more effective than CBT alone.

Medications

An international review of psychiatrists' management of patients with generalized anxiety disorder (GAD) reported that the preferred first-line pharmacological treatments of GAD were selective serotonin reuptake inhibitors (SSRIs) (80%), followed by serotonin–norepinephrine reuptake inhibitors (SNRIs) (43%), and pregabalin (35%). Preferred second-line treatments were SNRIs (41%) and pregabalin (36%).

Selective Serotonin Reuptake Inhibitors

Pharmaceutical treatments for GAD include selective serotonin reuptake inhibitors (SSRIs). These are the preferred first line of treatment. SSRIs used for this purpose include escitalopram and paroxetine.

Common side effects include nausea, sexual dysfunction, headache, diarrhea, constipation, restlessness, increased risk of suicide in young adults and adolescents, among others. Overdose of an SSRI can result in serotonin syndrome.

Benzodiazepines

Benzodiazepines are most often prescribed to patients with Generalized Anxiety Disorder. Research suggests that these drugs give some relief, at least in the short term. However, they carry some risks, mainly impairment of both cognitive and motor functioning, and psychological and physical dependence that makes it difficult for patients to stop taking them. It has been noted that people taking benzodiazepines are not as alert on their job or at school. Additionally, these drugs may impair driving and they are often associated with falls in the elderly, resulting in hip fractures. These shortcomings make the use of benzodiazepines optimal only for short-term relief of anxiety. CBT and medication are of comparable efficacy in the short-term but CBT has advantages over medication in the longer term.

Benzodiazepines (or "benzos") are fast-acting hypnotic sedatives that are also used to treat GAD and other anxiety disorders. Benzodiazepines are prescribed for generalized anxiety disorder and show beneficial effects in the short term. Popular Benzodiazepines for GAD include alprazolam, lorazepam and clonazepam. The World Council of Anxiety does not recommend the long-term use of benzodiazepines because they are associated with the development of tolerance, psychomotor impairment, cognitive and memory impairments, physical dependence and a withdrawal syndrome. Side effects include drowsiness, reduced motor coordination and problems with equilibrioception.

Pregabalin and Gabapentin

Pregabalin (Lyrica) acts on the voltage-dependent calcium channel to decrease the release of neurotransmitters such as glutamate, norepinephrine and substance P. Its therapeutic effect appears after 1 week of use and is similar in effectiveness to lorazepam, alprazolam and venlafaxine but pregabalin has demonstrated superiority by producing more consistent therapeutic effects for psychic and somatic anxiety symptoms. Long-term trials have shown continued effectiveness without the development of tolerance and additionally, unlike benzodiazepines, it does not disrupt sleep architecture and produces less severe cognitive and psychomotor impairment. It also has a low potential for abuse and dependency and may be preferred over the benzodiazepines for these reasons. The anxiolytic effects of pregabalin appear rapidly after administration, similar to the benzodiazepines, which gives pregabalin an advantage over many anxiolytic medications such as antidepressants.

Gabapentin (Neurontin), a closely related drug to pregabalin with the same mechanism of action, has also demonstrated effectiveness in the treatment of GAD, though unlike pregabalin, it has not been approved specifically for this indication. Nonetheless, it is likely to be of similar usefulness in the management of this condition, and by virtue of being off-patent, it has the advantage of being significantly less expensive in comparison. In accordance, gabapentin is frequently prescribed off-label to treat GAD.

Other Psychiatric Drugs

- 5-HT$_{1A}$ receptor partial agonists, such as buspirone and tandospirone.

- Serotonin-norepinephrine reuptake inhibitors (SNRIs), such as venlafaxine and duloxetine.

- Newer, atypical serotonergic antidepressants, such as vilazodone, vortioxetine, and agomelatine.

- Tricyclic antidepressants (TCAs), such as imipramine and clomipramine.

- Certain monoamine oxidase inhibitors (MAOIs), such as moclobemide and, rarely, phenelzine.

Other Drugs

- Hydroxyzine - Antihistamine, $5\text{-}HT_{2A}$ receptor antagonist.

- Propranolol - Sympatholytic, beta blocker.

- Clonidine - Sympatholytic, α_2-adrenergic receptor agonist.

- Guanfacine - Sympatholytic, α_2-adrenergic receptor agonist.

- Prazosin - Sympatholytic, alpha blocker.

Comorbidity

GAD and Depression

In the National Comorbidity Survey (2005), 58 percent of patients diagnosed with major depression were found to have an anxiety disorder; among these patients, the rate of comorbidity with GAD was 17.2 percent, and with panic disorder, 9.9 percent. Patients with a diagnosed anxiety disorder also had high rates of comorbid depression, including 22.4 percent of patients with social phobia, 9.4 percent with agoraphobia, and 2.3 percent with panic disorder. A longitudinal cohort study found 12% of the 972 participants had GAD comorbid with MDD. Accumulating evidence indicates that patients with comorbid depression and anxiety tend to have greater illness severity and a lower treatment response than those with either disorder alone. In addition, social function and quality of life are more greatly impaired.

For many, the symptoms of both depression and anxiety are not severe enough (i.e. are subsyndromal) to justify a primary diagnosis of either major depressive disorder (MDD) or an anxiety disorder. However, dysthymia is the most prevalent comorbid diagnosis of GAD clients. Patients can also be categorized as having mixed anxiety-depressive disorder, and they are at significantly increased risk of developing full-blown depression or anxiety.

GAD and Substance use Disorders

Those with GAD have a lifetime comorbidity prevalence of 30% to 35% with alcohol use disorder and 25% to 30% for another substance use disorder. People with both GAD and a substance use disorder also have a higher lifetime prevalence for other comorbidities. A study found that GAD was the primary disorder in slightly more than half of the 18 participants that were comorbid with alcohol use disorder.

Other Comorbidities

In addition to coexisting with depression, research shows that GAD often coexists with conditions associated with stress, such as irritable bowel syndrome. Patients with GAD can sometimes present with symptoms such as insomnia or headaches as well as pain, cardiac events and interpersonal problems.

Further research suggests that about 20 to 40 percent of individuals with attention deficit hyperactivity disorder have comorbid anxiety disorders, with GAD being the most prevalent.

The World Health Organization's Global Burden of Disease project did not include generalized anxiety disorders. In lieu of global statistics, here are some prevalence rates from around the world:

- Australia: 3 percent of adults
- Canada: Between 3 and 5 percent of adults
- Italy: 2.9 percent
- Taiwan: 0.4 percent
- United States: approx. 3.1 percent of people age 18 and over in a given year (9.5 million)

The usual age of onset is variable, from childhood to late adulthood, with the median age of onset being approximately 31 and mean age of onset is 32.7. Most studies find that GAD is associated with an earlier and more gradual onset than the other anxiety disorders. The prevalence of GAD in children is approximately 3%; the prevalence in adolescents is reported as high as 10.8%. When GAD appears in children and adolescents, it typically begins around 8 to 9 years of age.

Populations with a higher rate of diagnosis of GAD are individuals that are traditionally oppressed. This includes individuals with low and middle socio-economic status, separated, divorced, and widowed individuals. Women are twice as likely to develop GAD as men. This is primarily because women are more likely than men to live in poverty, be subject to discrimination, and be sexually and physically abused. African Americans have significantly higher odds of enduring GAD and the disorder often manifests itself in different patterns. Other populations that are more diagnosed with GAD are those who live alone, those with a low level of education, and the unemployed. GAD is also common in the elderly population.

Compared to the general population, patients with internalizing disorders such as depression, generalized anxiety disorder (GAD) and post-traumatic stress disorder (PTSD) have higher mortality rates, but die of the same age-related diseases as the population, such as heart disease, cerebrovascular disease and cancer.

Comorbidity and Treatment

A study on comorbidity of GAD and other depressive disorders has shown that treatment is not more or less effective when there is some sort of comorbidity of another disorder. The severity of symptoms did not affect the outcome of the treatment process in these cases.

Generalized Anxiety Disorder 7

Generalized Anxiety Disorder 7 (GAD-7) is a self-reported questionnaire for screening and severity measuring of generalized anxiety disorder (GAD). GAD-7 has seven items, which measure severity of various signs of GAD according to reported response categories with assigned points. Assessment is indicated by the total score, which made up by adding together the scores for the scale all seven items.

GAD-7 is a sensitive self-administrated test to assess generalized anxiety disorder, normally used in outpatient and primary care settings for referral to psychiatrist pending outcome. However, it cannot be used as replacement for clinical assessment and additional evaluation should be used to confirm a diagnosis of GAD.

The scale uses a normative system of scoring as shown below - [bullet points of answer options and points assigned] - with question at the end qualitatively describing severity of the patient's anxiety over the past 2 weeks.

- Not at all (0 points)

- Several days (1 point)

- More than half the days (2 points)

- Nearly every day (3 points)

References

- Diagnostic and Statistical Manual of Mental DisordersAmerican Psychiatric Associati. (5th ed.). Arlington: American Psychiatric Publishing. 2013. pp. 189–195. ISBN 978-0890425558

- Stein, MB; Sareen, J (19 November 2015). "Clinical Practice: Generalized Anxiety Disorder.". The New England Journal of Medicine. 373 (21): 2059–68. PMID 26580998. doi:10.1056/nejmcp1502514

- "Adult Separation Anxiety Often Overlooked Diagnosis – Arehart-Treichel 41 (13): 30 – Psychiatr News". Psychiatric News. Retrieved 20 February 2012

- Neal, Angela M.; Turner, Samuel M. (May 1991). "Anxiety disorders research with African Americans: Current status". Psychological Bulletin. 109 (3): 400–410. doi:10.1037/0033-2909.109.3.400

- Evans, Katie; Sullivan, Michael J. (1 March 2001). Dual Diagnosis: Counseling the Mentally Ill Substance Abuser (2nd ed.). Guilford Press. pp. 75–76. ISBN 978-1-57230-446-8

- Kozlowska K.; Hanney L. (1999). "Family assessment and intervention using an interactive are exercise". Australia and New Zealand Journal of Family Therapy. 20 (2): 61–69. doi:10.1002/j.1467-8438.1999.tb00358.x

- Warren Mansell (1 June 2007). "Reading about self-help books on cognitive-behavioural therapy for anxiety disorders". Pb.rcpsych.org. Retrieved 20 February 2012

- Durham, Rob C. (2007). "Treatment of generalized anxiety disorder". Psychiatry. 6 (5): 183–187. doi:10.1016/j.mppsy.2007.03.003

- Lindsay, S.J.E.; Powell, Graham E., eds. (28 July 1998). The Handbook of Clinical Adult Psychology (2nd ed.). Routledge. pp. 152–153. ISBN 978-0-415-07215-1

- Schneier, Franklin (7 September 2006). "Social Anxiety Disorder". The New England Journal of Medicine. 355: 1029–1036. PMID 16957148. doi:10.1056/nejmcp060145

- Cloos, Jean-Marc (2005). "The Treatment of Panic Disorder". Curr Opin Psychiatry. 18 (1): 45–50. PMID 16639183. Retrieved 25 September 2007

- Craske, MG; Stein, MB (24 June 2016). "Anxiety.". Lancet (London, England). PMID 27349358. doi:10.1016/S0140-6736(16)30381-6

- American Psychiatric Association (2013). Diagnostic and Statistical Manual of Mental Disorders (DSM-5). American Psychiatric Publishing. pp. 226–230. ISBN 978-0-89042-555-8

- Katzelnick, D. J.; Greist, J. H. (2001). "Social anxiety disorder: An unrecognized problem in primary care". The Journal of Clinical Psychiatry. 62 Suppl 1: 11–15; discussion 15–6. PMID 11206029

- "Clinical guidelines and evidence review for panic disorder and generalised anxiety disorder" (PDF). National Collaborating Centre for Primary Care. 2004. Retrieved 16 June 2009

- Jurbergs N. Ledley (2005). "Separation anxiety disorder". Pediatric Annals. 34 (2): 108–15. doi:10.3928/0090-4481-20050201-09

- World Health Organization (2009). Pharmacological Treatment of Mental Disorders in Primary Health Care (PDF). Geneva. ISBN 978-92-4-154769-7

- Agoraphobia Resource Center. "Agoraphobia treatments—Eye movement desensitization and reprogramming". Archived from the original on 5 April 2008. Retrieved 2008-04-18

- Rapee R. M.; Spence S. H. (2004). "The etiology of social phobia: empirical evidence and an initial model". Clin Psychol Rev. 24 (7): 737–767. PMID 15501555. doi:10.1016/j.cpr.2004.06.004

Mood Disorder: Therapies

Cognitive behavioral therapy is a form of psychosocial treatment that helps in altering undesired thoughts and habits. It has been shown to be effective in treating milder forms of anxiety and depression disorders, substance abuse problems and posttraumatic stress disorder. The aspects elucidated in this chapter are of vital importance, and provide a better understanding of mood disorders.

Cognitive Behavioral Therapy

Cognitive behavioral therapy (CBT) is a psychosocial intervention that is the most widely used evidence-based practice for treating mental disorders. Guided by empirical research, CBT focuses on the development of personal coping strategies that target solving current problems and changing unhelpful patterns in cognitions (e.g. thoughts, beliefs, and attitudes), behaviors, and emotional regulation. It was originally designed to treat depression, and is now used for a number of mental health conditions.

The CBT model is based on a combination of the basic principles from behavioral and cognitive psychology. It is different from historical approaches to psychotherapy, such as the psychoanalytic approach where the therapist looks for the unconscious meaning behind behaviors and then formulates a diagnosis. Instead, CBT is "problem-focused" and "action-oriented", meaning it is used to treat specific problems related to a diagnosed mental disorder and the therapist's role is to assist the client in finding and practising effective strategies to address the identified goals and decrease symptoms of the disorder. CBT is based on the belief that thought distortions and maladaptive behaviors play a role in the development and maintenance of psychological disorders, and that symptoms and associated distress can be reduced by teaching new information-processing skills and coping mechanisms.

When compared to psychotropic medications, review studies have found CBT-alone to be as effective for treating less severe forms of depression and anxiety, posttraumatic stress disorder (PTSD), tics, substance abuse (with the exception of opioid use disorder), eating disorders, and borderline personality disorder, and it is often recommended in combination with medications for treating other conditions, such as severe obsessive compulsive disorder (OCD) and Major depressive disorder, opioid addiction, bipolar, and psychotic disorders. In addition, CBT is recommended as the first line of treatment for the majority of psychological disorders in children and adolescents, including aggression and conduct disorder. Researchers have found that other *bona fide* therapeutic interventions were equally effective for treating certain conditions in adults, but CBT was found to be superior in treating most disorders. Along with interpersonal psychotherapy (IPT), CBT is recommended in treatment guidelines as a psychosocial treatment of choice, and CBT and IPT are the only psychosocial interventions that psychiatry residents are mandated to be trained in.

Description

Mainstream cognitive behavioral therapy assumes that changing maladaptive thinking leads to change in behavior and affect, but recent variants emphasize changes in one's relationship to maladaptive thinking rather than changes in thinking itself. The goal of cognitive behavioral therapy is not to diagnose a person with a particular disease, but to look at the person as a whole and decide what needs to be fixed. The basic steps in a cognitive-behavioral assessment include:

Step 1: Identify critical behaviors

Step 2: Determine whether critical behaviors are excesses or deficits

Step 3: Evaluate critical behaviors for frequency, duration, or intensity (obtain a baseline)

Step 4: If excess, attempt to decrease frequency, duration, or intensity of behaviors; if deficits, attempt to increase behaviors.

These steps are based on a system created by Kanfer and Saslow. After identifying the behaviors that need changing, whether they be in excess or deficit, and treatment has occurred, the psychologist must identify whether or not the intervention succeeded. For example, "If the goal was to decrease the behavior, then there should be a decrease relative to the baseline. If the critical behavior remains at or above the baseline, then the intervention has failed."

Therapists or computer-based programs use CBT techniques to help individuals challenge their patterns and beliefs and replace "errors in thinking such as overgeneralizing, magnifying negatives, minimizing positives and catastrophizing" with "more realistic and effective thoughts, thus decreasing emotional distress and self-defeating behavior." These errors in thinking are known as cognitive distortions. Cognitive distortions can be either a pseudo-discrimination belief or an over-generalization of something. CBT techniques may also be used to help individuals take a more open, mindful, and aware posture toward cognitive distortions so as to diminish their impact. Mainstream CBT helps individuals replace "maladaptive... coping skills, cognitions, emotions and behaviors with more adaptive ones", by challenging an individual's way of thinking and the way that they react to certain habits or behaviors, but there is still controversy about the degree to which these traditional cognitive elements account for the effects seen with CBT over and above the earlier behavioral elements such as exposure and skills training.

Modern forms of CBT include a variety of diverse but related techniques such as expo-sure therapy, stress inoculation, cognitive processing therapy, cognitive therapy, re-laxation training, dialectical behavior therapy, and acceptance and commitment ther-apy. Some practitioners promote a form of mindful cognitive therapy which includes a greater emphasis on self-awareness as part of the therapeutic process.

CBT has six phases:

1. Assessment or psychological assessment;

2. Reconceptualization;

3. Skills acquisition;

4. Skills consolidation and application training;

5. Generalization and maintenance;

6. Post-treatment assessment follow-up.

The reconceptualization phase makes up much of the "cognitive" portion of CBT. A summary of modern CBT approaches is given by Hofmann.

There are different protocols for delivering cognitive behavioral therapy, with import-ant similarities among them. Use of the term *CBT* may refer to different interventions, including "self-instructions (e.g. distraction, imagery, motivational self-talk), relax-ation and/or biofeedback, development of adaptive coping strategies (e.g. minimizing negative or self-defeating thoughts), changing maladaptive beliefs about pain, and goal setting". Treatment is sometimes manualized, with brief, direct, and time-limited treat-ments for individual psychological disorders that are specific technique-driven. CBT is used in both individual and group settings, and the techniques are often adapted for self-help applications. Some clinicians and researchers are cognitively oriented (e.g. cognitive restructuring), while others are more behaviorally oriented (e.g. *in vivo* ex-posure therapy). Interventions such as imaginal exposure therapy combine both ap-proaches.

Medical Uses

In adults, CBT has been shown to have effectiveness and a role in the treatment plans for anxiety disorders, depression, eating disorders, chronic low back pain, personal-ity disorders, psychosis, schizophrenia, substance use disorders, in the adjustment, depression, and anxiety associated with fibromyalgia, and with post-spinal cord in-juries.

In children or adolescents, CBT is an effective part of treatment plans for anxiety disor-ders, body dysmorphic disorder, depression and suicidality, eating disorders and obe-sity, obsessive–compulsive disorder (OCD), and posttraumatic stress disorder, as well as tic disorders, trichotillomania, and other repetitive behavior disorders. CBT-SP, an adaptation of CBT for suicide prevention (SP), was specifically designed for treating youths who are severely depressed and who have recently attempted suicide within the past 90 days, and was found to be effective, feasible, and acceptable. *Sparx* is a video game to help young persons, using the CBT method to teach them how to resolve their own issues. CBT has also been shown to be effective for posttraumatic stress disorder in very young children (3 to 6 years of age). CBT has also been applied to a variety of childhood disorders, including depressive disorders and various anxiety disorders.

Cochrane reviews have found no evidence that CBT is effective for tinnitus, although there appears to be an effect on management of associated depression and quality of life in this condition. Other recent Cochrane Reviews found no convincing evidence that CBT training helps foster care providers manage difficult behaviors in the youths under their care, nor was it helpful in treating people who abuse their intimate partners.

According to a 2004 review by INSERM of three methods, cognitive behavioral therapy was either "proven" or "presumed" to be an effective therapy on several specific mental disorders. According to the study, CBT was effective at treating schizophrenia, depression, bipolar disorder, panic disorder, post-traumatic stress, anxiety disorders, bulimia, anorexia, personality disorders and alcohol dependency.

Some meta-analyses find CBT more effective than psychodynamic therapy and equal to other therapies in treating anxiety and depression.

Computerized CBT (CCBT) has been proven to be effective by randomized controlled and other trials in treating depression and anxiety disorders, including children, as well as insomnia. Some research has found similar effectiveness to an intervention of informational websites and weekly telephone calls. CCBT was found to be equally effective as face-to-face CBT in adolescent anxiety and insomnia.

Criticism of CBT sometimes focuses on implementations (such as the UK IAPT) which may result initially in low quality therapy being offered by poorly trained practitioners. However evidence supports the effectiveness of CBT for anxiety and depression.

Mounting evidence suggests that the addition of hypnotherapy as an adjunct to CBT improves treatment efficacy for a variety of clinical issues.

CBT has been applied in both clinical and non-clinical environments to treat disorders such as personality conditions and behavioral problems. A systematic review of CBT in depression and anxiety disorders concluded that "CBT delivered in primary care, especially including computer- or Internet-based self-help programs, is potentially more effective than usual care and could be delivered effectively by primary care therapists."

Emerging evidence suggests a possible role for CBT in the treatment of attention deficit hyperactivity disorder (ADHD); hypochondriasis; coping with the impact of multiple sclerosis; sleep disturbances related to aging; dysmenorrhea; and bipolar disorder, but more study is needed and results should be interpreted with caution. CBT can have a therapeutic effects on easing symptoms of anxiety and depression in people with Alzheimer's disease. CBT has been studied as an aid in the treatment of anxiety associated with stuttering. Initial studies have shown CBT to be effective in reducing social anxiety in adults who stutter, but not in reducing stuttering frequency.

In the case of people with metastatic breast cancer, data is limited but CBT and other psychosocial interventions might help with psychological outcomes and pain management.

There is some evidence that CBT is superior in the long-term to benzodiazepines and the nonbenzodiazepines in the treatment and management of insomnia. CBT has been shown to be moderately effective for treating chronic fatigue syndrome.

In the United Kingdom, the National Institute for Health and Care Excellence (NICE) recommends CBT in the treatment plans for a number of mental health difficulties, including posttraumatic stress disorder, obsessive–compulsive disorder (OCD), bulimia nervosa, and clinical depression.

Anxiety Disorders

CBT has been shown to be effective in the treatment of adult anxiety disorders.

A basic concept in some CBT treatments used in anxiety disorders is *in vivo* exposure. The term refers to the direct confrontation of feared objects, activities, or situations by a patient. For example, a woman with PTSD who fears the location where she was assaulted may be assisted by her therapist in going to that location and directly confronting those fears. Likewise, a person with social anxiety disorder who fears public speaking may be instructed to directly confront those fears by giving a speech. This "two-factor" model is often credited to O. Hobart Mowrer. Through exposure to the stimulus, this harmful conditioning can be "unlearned" (referred to as extinction and habituation). Studies have provided evidence that when examining animals and humans that glucocorticoids may possibly lead to a more successful extinction learning during exposure therapy. For instance, glucocorticoids can prevent aversive learning episodes from being retrieved and heighten reinforcement of memory traces creating a non-fearful reaction in feared situations. A combination of glucocorticoids and exposure therapy may be a better improved treatment for treating patients with anxiety disorders.

Schizophrenia, Psychosis and Mood Disorders

Cognitive behavioral therapy has been shown as an effective treatment for clinical depression. The American Psychiatric Association Practice Guidelines (April 2000) indicated that, among psychotherapeutic approaches, cognitive behavioral therapy and interpersonal psychotherapy had the best-documented efficacy for treatment of major depressive disorder. One etiological theory of depression is Aaron T. Beck's cognitive theory of depression. His theory states that depressed people think the way they do because their thinking is biased towards negative interpretations. According to this theory, depressed people acquire a negative schema of the world in childhood and adolescence as an effect of stressful life events, and the negative schema is activated later in life when the person encounters similar situations.

Beck also described a negative cognitive triad, made up of the negative schemata and cognitive biases of the person, theorizing that depressed individuals make negative evaluations of themselves, the world, and the future. According to this theory, depressed people have views such as "I never do a good job", "It is impossible to have a good day", and "things will never get better." A negative schema helps give rise to the cognitive bias, and the cognitive bias helps fuel the negative schema. This is the negative triad. Beck further proposed that depressed people often have the following cognitive biases: arbitrary inference, selective abstraction, over-generalization, magnification, and minimization. These cognitive biases are quick to make negative, generalized, and personal inferences of the self, thus fueling the negative schema.

In long-term psychoses, CBT is used to complement medication and is adapted to meet individual needs. Interventions particularly related to these conditions include exploring reality testing, changing delusions and hallucinations, examining factors which precipitate relapse, and managing relapses. Several meta-analyses suggested that CBT is effective in schizophrenia, and the American Psychiatric Association includes CBT in its schizophrenia guideline as an evidence-based treatment. There is also limited evidence of effectiveness for CBT in bipolar disorder and severe depression.

A 2010 meta-analysis found that no trial employing both blinding and psychological placebo has shown CBT to be effective in either schizophrenia or bipolar disorder, and that the effect size of CBT was small in major depressive disorder. They also found a lack of evidence to conclude that CBT was effective in preventing relapses in bipolar disorder. Evidence that severe depression is mitigated by CBT is also lacking, with anti-depressant medications still viewed as significantly more effective than CBT, although success with CBT for depression was observed beginning in the 1990s.

According to Cox, Abramson, Devine, and Hollon (2012), cognitive behavioral therapy can also be used to reduce prejudice towards others. This other-directed prejudice can cause depression in the "others," or in the self when a person becomes part of a group he or she previously had prejudice towards (i.e. deprejudice). "Devine and colleagues (2012) developed a successful Prejudice Perpetrator intervention with many conceptual parallels to CBT. Like CBT, their intervention taught Sources to be aware of their automative thoughts and to intentionally deploy a variety of cognitive techniques against automatic stereotyping."

Comparison of CBT to other psychosocial treatments for schizophrenia			
Measured outcome	**Findings in words**	**Findings in numbers**	**Quality of evidence**
Global effects			
No change in mental state	CBT seems no better than other psychosocial treatments for mental state	RR 0.84 CI 0.64 to 1.09	Very low
Relapse	Relapse was not reduced by CBT	RR 0.91 CI 0.63 to 1.32	Low
Rehospitalisation	Rehospitalisation was not reduced by CBT	RR 0.86 CI 0.62 to 1.21	Low
Social functioning	Social functioning was improved in the CBT group - at about 26 weeks - but it is unclear what this means in everyday life	MD 8.80 higher CI 4.07 to 21.67	Very low
High quality of life	Quality of life was not changed in the CBT group	MD 1.86 lower CI 19.2 lower to 15.48 higher	Very low
Adverse effects			
Adverse effects (within 24–52 weeks of onset of therapy)	No more likely to have adverse effects with CBT	RR 2 CI 0.71 to 5.64	Very low

With Older Adults

CBT is used to help people of all ages, but the therapy should be adjusted based on the age of the patient with whom the therapist is dealing. Older individuals in particular have certain characteristics that need to be acknowledged and the therapy altered to account for these differences thanks to age.

Prevention of Mental Illness

For anxiety disorders, use of CBT with people at risk has significantly reduced the number of episodes of generalized anxiety disorder and other anxiety symptoms, and also given significant improvements in explanatory style, hopelessness, and dysfunctional attitudes. In another study, 3% of the group receiving the CBT intervention developed generalized anxiety disorder by 12 months postintervention compared with 14% in the control group. Subthreshold panic disorder sufferers were found to significantly benefit from use of CBT. Use of CBT was found to significantly reduce social anxiety prevalence.

For depressive disorders, a stepped-care intervention (watchful waiting, CBT and medication if appropriate) achieved a 50% lower incidence rate in a patient group aged 75 or older. Another depression study found a neutral effect compared to personal, social, and health education, and usual school provision, and included a comment on potential for increased depression scores from people who have received CBT due to greater self recognition and acknowledgement of existing symptoms of depression and negative thinking styles. A further study also saw a neutral result. A meta-study of the Coping with Depression course, a cognitive behavioral intervention delivered by a psychoeducational method, saw a 38% reduction in risk of major depression.

For people at risk of psychosis, in 2014 the UK National Institute for Health and Care Excellence (NICE) recommended preventive CBT.

Gambling Addiction

CBT is also used for problem gambling addiction. The number of individuals who gamble is 1–3% around the world. Cognitive behavioral therapy develop skills for relapse prevention and learn to control mind and manage high-risk cases.

History

Philosophical roots

Precursors of certain fundamental aspects of CBT have been identified in various ancient philosophical traditions, particularly Stoicism. Stoic philosophers, particularly Epictetus, believed logic could be used to identify and discard false beliefs that lead to destructive emotions, which has influenced the way modern cognitive-behavioral therapists identify cognitive distortions that contribute to depression and anxiety. For example, Aaron T. Beck's original treatment manual for depression states, "The philosophical origins of cognitive therapy can be traced back to the Stoic philosophers". Another example of Stoic influence on cognitive theorists is Epictetus on Albert Ellis. A key philosophical figure who also influenced the development of CBT was John Stuart Mill.

Behavior Therapy Roots

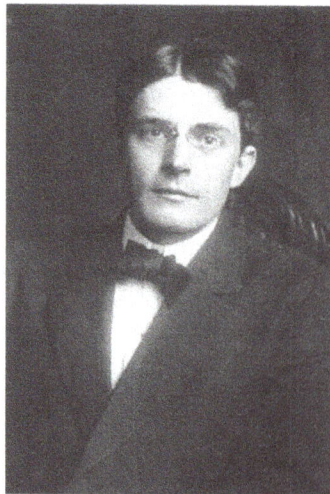

John B. Watson

The modern roots of CBT can be traced to the development of behavior therapy in the early

20th century, the development of cognitive therapy in the 1960s, and the subsequent merging of the two. Groundbreaking work of behaviorism began with John B. Watson and Rosalie Rayner's studies of conditioning in 1920. Behaviorally-centered therapeutic approaches appeared as early as 1924 with Mary Cover Jones' work dedicated to the unlearning of fears in children. These were the antecedents of the development of Joseph Wolpe's behavioral therapy in the 1950s. It was the work of Wolpe and Watson, which was based on Ivan Pavlov's work on learning and conditioning, that influenced Hans Eysenck and Arnold Lazarus to develop new behavioral therapy techniques based on classical conditioning. One of Eysenck's colleagues, Glenn Wilson showed that classical fear conditioning in humans could be controlled by verbally induced cognitive expectations, thus opening a field of research that supports the rationale of cognitive behaviorial therapy.

During the 1950s and 1960s, behavioral therapy became widely utilized by researchers in the United States, the United Kingdom, and South Africa, who were inspired by the behaviorist learning theory of Ivan Pavlov, John B. Watson, and Clark L. Hull. In Britain, Joseph Wolpe, who applied the findings of animal experiments to his method of systematic desensitization, applied behavioral research to the treatment of neurotic disorders. Wolpe's therapeutic efforts were precursors to today's fear reduction techniques. British psychologist Hans Eysenck presented behavior therapy as a constructive alternative.

At the same time of Eysenck's work, B. F. Skinner and his associates were beginning to have an impact with their work on operant conditioning. Skinner's work was referred to as radical behaviorism and avoided anything related to cognition. However, Julian Rotter, in 1954, and Albert Bandura, in 1969, contributed behavior therapy with their respective work on social learning theory, by demonstrating the effects of cognition on learning and behavior modification.

The emphasis on behavioral factors constituted the "first wave" of CBT.

Cognitive Therapy Roots

One of the first therapists to address cognition in psychotherapy was Alfred Adler with his notion of basic mistakes and how they contributed to creation of unhealthy or useless behavioral and life goals. Adler's work influenced the work of Albert Ellis, who developed one of the earliest cognitive-based psychotherapies, known today as Rational emotive behavior therapy, or REBT.

Around the same time that rational emotive therapy, as it was known then, was being developed, Aaron T. Beck was conducting free association sessions in his psychoanalytic practice. During these sessions, Beck noticed that thoughts were not as unconscious as Freud had previously theorized, and that certain types of thinking may be the culprits of emotional distress. It was from this hypothesis that Beck developed cognitive therapy, and called these thoughts "automatic thoughts".

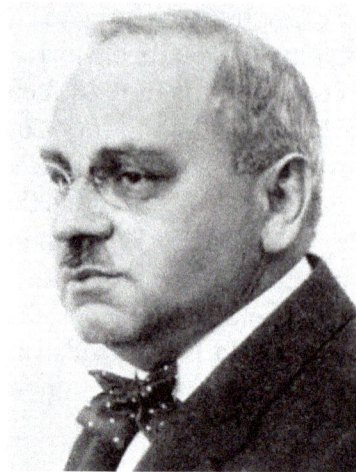

Alfred Adler

It was these two therapies, rational emotive therapy and cognitive therapy, that started the "second wave" of CBT, which was the emphasis on cognitive factors.

Behavior and Cognitive Therapies Merge

Although the early behavioral approaches were successful in many of the neurotic disorders, they had little success in treating depression. Behaviorism was also losing in popularity due to the so-called "cognitive revolution". The therapeutic approaches of Albert Ellis and Aaron T. Beck gained popularity among behavior therapists, despite the earlier behaviorist rejection of "mentalistic" concepts like thoughts and cognitions. Both of these systems included behavioral elements and interventions and primarily concentrated on problems in the present.

In initial studies, cognitive therapy was often contrasted with behavioral treatments to see which was most effective. During the 1980s and 1990s, cognitive and behavioral techniques were merged into cognitive behavioral therapy. Pivotal to this merging was the successful development of treatments for panic disorder by David M. Clark in the UK and David H. Barlow in the US.

Over time, cognitive behavior therapy became to be known not only as a therapy, but as an umbrella term for all cognitive-based psychotherapies. These therapies include, but are not limited to, rational emotive therapy, cognitive therapy, acceptance and commitment therapy, dialectical behavior therapy, reality therapy/choice theory, cognitive processing therapy, EMDR, and multimodal therapy. All of these therapies are a blending of cognitive- and behavior-based elements.

This blending of theoretical and technical foundations from both behavior and cognitive therapies constitute the "third wave" of CBT, which is the current wave. The most prominent therapies of this third wave are dialectical behavior therapy and acceptance and commitment therapy.

Methods of Access

Therapist

A typical CBT programme would consist of face-to-face sessions between patient and therapist, made up of 6-18 sessions of around an hour each with a gap of a 1–3 weeks between sessions. This initial programme might be followed by some booster sessions, for instance after one month and three months. CBT has also been found to be effective if patient and therapist type in real time to each other over computer links.

Cognitive behavioral therapy is most closely allied with the scientist–practitioner model in which clinical practice and research is informed by a scientific perspective, clear operationalization of the problem, and an emphasis on measurement, including measuring changes in cognition and behavior and in the attainment of goals. These are often met through "homework" assignments in which the patient and the therapist work together to craft an assignment to complete before the next session. The completion of these assignments – which can be as simple as a person suffering from depression attending some kind of social event – indicates a dedication to treatment compliance and a desire to change. The therapists can then logically gauge the next step of treatment based on how thoroughly the patient completes the assignment. Effective cognitive behavioral therapy is dependent on a therapeutic alliance between the healthcare practitioner and the person seeking assistance. Unlike many other forms of psychotherapy, the patient is very involved in CBT. For example, an anxious patient may be asked to talk to a stranger as a homework assignment, but if that is too difficult, he or she can work out an easier assignment first. The therapist needs to be flexible and willing to listen to the patient rather than acting as an authority figure.

Computerized or Internet-delivered

Computerized cognitive behavioral therapy (CCBT) has been described by NICE as a *"generic term for delivering CBT via an interactive computer interface delivered by a personal computer, internet, or interactive voice response system"*, instead of face-to-face with a human therapist. It is also known as internet-delivered cognitive behavioral therapy or ICBT. CCBT has potential to improve access to evidence-based therapies, and to overcome the prohibitive costs and lack of availability sometimes associated with retaining a human therapist. In this context, it is important not to confuse CBT with 'computer-based training', which nowadays is more commonly referred to as e-Learning.

CCBT has been found in meta-studies to be cost-effective and often cheaper than usual care, including for anxiety. Studies have shown that individuals with social anxiety and depression experienced improvement with online CBT-based methods. A review of current CCBT research in the treatment of OCD in children found this interface to hold great potential for future treatment of OCD in youths and adolescent populations.

CCBT is also predisposed to treating mood disorders amongst non-heterosexual populations, who may avoid face-to-face therapy from fear of stigma. However presently CCBT programs seldom cater to these populations.

A key issue in CCBT use is low uptake and completion rates, even when it has been clearly made available and explained. CCBT completion rates and treatment efficacy have been found in some studies to be higher when use of CCBT is supported personally, with supporters not limited only to therapists, than when use is in a self-help form alone. Another approach to improving uptake and completion rate, as well as treatment outcome, is to design software that supports the formation of a strong therapeutic alliance between the user and the technology.

In February 2006 NICE recommended that CCBT be made available for use within the NHS across England and Wales for patients presenting with mild-to-moderate depression, rather than immediately opting for antidepressant medication, and CCBT is made available by some health systems. The 2009 NICE guideline recognized that there are likely to be a number of computerized CBT products that are useful to patients, but removed endorsement of any specific product.

A relatively new avenue of research is the combination of artificial intelligence and CCBT. It has been proposed to use modern technology to create CCBT that simulates face-to-face therapy. This might be achieved in cognitive behavior therapy for a specific disorder using the comprehensive domain knowledge of CBT. One area where this has been attempted is the specific domain area of social anxiety in those who stutter.

Reading self-help Materials

Enabling patients to read self-help CBT guides has been shown to be effective by some studies. However one study found a negative effect in patients who tended to ruminate, and another meta-analysis found that the benefit was only significant when the self-help was guided (e.g. by a medical professional).

Group Educational Course

Patient participation in group courses has been shown to be effective. In a meta-analysis reviewing evidence-based treatment of OCD in children, individual CBT was found to be more efficacious than group CBT.

Types

Brief CBT

Brief cognitive behavioral therapy (BCBT) is a form of CBT which has been developed for situations in which there are time constraints on the therapy sessions. BCBT takes place over a couple of sessions that can last up to 12 accumulated hours by design. This technique was first implemented and developed on soldiers overseas in active duty by David M. Rudd to prevent suicide.

Breakdown of treatment

1. Orientation

    1. Commitment to treatment

    2. Crisis response and safety planning

    3. Means restriction

    4. Survival kit

    5. Reasons for living card

    6. Model of suicidality

    7. Treatment journal

    8. Lessons learned

2. Skill focus

    1. Skill development worksheets

    2. Coping cards

    3. Demonstration

    4. Practice

    5. Skill refinement

3. Relapse prevention

    1. Skill generalization

    2. Skill refinement

Cognitive Emotional Behavioral Therapy

Cognitive emotional behavioral therapy (CEBT) is a form of CBT developed initially for individuals with eating disorders but now used with a range of problems including anxiety, depression, obsessive compulsive disorder (OCD), post-traumatic stress disorder (PTSD) and anger problems. It combines aspects of CBT and dialectical behavioral therapy and aims to improve understanding and tolerance of emotions in order to facilitate the therapeutic process. It is frequently used as a "pretreatment" to prepare and better equip individuals for longer-term therapy.

Structured Cognitive Behavioral Training

Structured cognitive behavioral training (SCBT) is a cognitive-based process with core philosophies that draw heavily from CBT. Like CBT, SCBT asserts that behavior is inextricably related to beliefs, thoughts and emotions. SCBT also builds on core CBT philosophy by incorporating other well-known modalities in the fields of behavioral health and psychology: most notably, Albert Ellis's Rational Emotive Behavior Therapy. SCBT differs from CBT in two distinct ways. First, SCBT is delivered in a highly regimented format. Second, SCBT is a predetermined and finite training process that becomes personalized by the input of the participant. SCBT is designed with the intention to bring a participant to a specific result in a specific period of time. SCBT has been used to challenge addictive behavior, particularly with substances such as tobacco, alcohol and food, and to manage diabetes and subdue stress and anxiety. SCBT has also been used in the field of criminal psychology in the effort to reduce recidivism.

Moral Reconation Therapy

Moral reconation therapy, a type of CBT used to help felons overcome antisocial personality disorder (ASPD), slightly decreases the risk of further offending. It is generally implemented in a group format because of the risk of offenders with ASPD being given one-on-one therapy reinforces narcissistic behavioral characteristics, and can be used in correctional or outpatient settings. Groups usually meet weekly for two to six months.

Stress Inoculation Training

This type of therapy uses a blend of cognitive, behavioral and some humanistic training techniques to target the stressors of the client. This usually is used to help clients better cope with their stress or anxiety after stressful events. This is a three-phase process that trains the client to use skills that they already have to better adapt to their current stressors. The first phase is an interview phase that includes psychological testing, client self-monitoring, and a variety of reading materials. This allows the therapist to individually tailor the training process to the client. Clients learn how to categorize problems into emotion-focused or problem-focused, so that they can better treat their negative situations. This phase ultimately prepares the client to eventually confront and reflect upon their current reactions to stressors, before looking at ways to change their reactions and emotions in relation to their stressors. The focus is conceptualization.

The second phase emphasizes the aspect of skills acquisition and rehearsal that continues from the earlier phase of conceptualization. The client is taught skills that help them cope with their stressors. These skills are then practised in the space of therapy. These skills involve self-regulation, problem-solving, interpersonal communication skills, etc.

The third and final phase is the application and following through of the skills learned in the training process. This gives the client opportunities to apply their learned skills to a wide range of stressors. Activities include role-playing, imagery, modeling, etc. In the end, the client will have been trained on a preventative basis to inoculate personal, chronic, and future stressors by breaking down their stressors into problems they will address in long-term, short-term, and intermediate coping goals.

Criticisms

Relative Effectiveness

The research conducted for CBT has been a topic of sustained controversy. While some researchers write that CBT is more effective than other treatments, many other researchers and practitioners have questioned the validity of such claims. For example, one study determined CBT to be superior to other treatments in treating anxiety and depression. However, researchers responding directly to that study conducted a re-analysis and found no evidence of CBT being superior to other bona fide treatments, and conducted an analysis of thirteen other CBT clinical trials and determined that they failed to provide evidence of CBT superiority.

A major criticism has been that clinical studies of CBT efficacy (or any psychotherapy) are not double-blind (i.e., either the subjects or the therapists in psychotherapy studies are not blind to the type of treatment). They may be single-blinded, i.e. the rater may not know the treatment the patient received, but neither the patients nor the therapists are blinded to the type of therapy given (two out of three of the persons involved in the trial, i.e., all of the persons involved in the treatment, are unblinded). The patient is an active participant in correcting negative distorted thoughts, thus quite aware of the treatment group they are in.

The importance of double-blinding was shown in a meta-analysis that examined the effectiveness of CBT when placebo control and blindedness were factored in. Pooled data from published trials of CBT in schizophrenia, major depressive disorder (MDD), and bipolar disorder that used controls for non-specific effects of intervention were analyzed. This study concluded that CBT is no better than non-specific control interventions in the treatment of schizophrenia and does not reduce relapse rates; treatment effects are small in treatment studies of MDD, and it is not an effective treatment strategy for prevention of relapse in bipolar disorder. For MDD, the authors note that the pooled effect size was very low. Nevertheless, the methodological processes used to select the studies in the previously mentioned meta-analysis and the worth of its findings have been called into question.

Declining Effectiveness

Additionally, a 2015 meta-analysis revealed that the positive effects of CBT on depression have been declining since 1977. The overall results showed two different declines in effect sizes: 1) an overall decline between 1977 and 2014, and 2) a steeper decline between 1995 and 2014. Additional sub-analysis revealed that CBT studies where therapists in the test group were instructed to adhere to the Beck CBT manual had a steeper decline in effect sizes since 1977 than studies where therapists in the test group were instructed to use CBT without a manual. The authors reported that they were unsure why the effects were declining but did list inadequate therapist training, failure to adhere to a manual, lack of therapist experience, and patients' hope and faith in its efficacy waning as potential reasons. The authors did mention that the current study was limited to depressive disorders only.

High drop-out Rates

Furthermore, other researchers write that CBT studies have high drop-out rates compared to other treatments. At times, the CBT drop-out rates can be more than five times higher than other treatments groups. For example, the researchers provided statistics of 28 participants in a group receiving CBT therapy dropping out, compared to 5 participants in a group receiving problem-solving therapy dropping out, or 11 participants in a group receiving psychodynamic therapy dropping out. This high drop-out rate is also evident in the treatment of several disorders, particularly the eating disorder anorexia nervosa, which is commonly treated with CBT. Those treated with CBT have a high chance of dropping out of therapy before completion and reverting to their anorexia behaviors.

Other researchers conducting an analysis of treatments for youths who self-injure found similar drop-out rates in CBT and DBT groups. In this study, the researchers analyzed several clinical trials that measured the efficacy of CBT administered to youths who self-injure. The researchers concluded that none of them were found to be efficacious. These conclusions were made using the APA Division 12 Task Force on the Promotion and Dissemination of Psychological Procedures to determine intervention potency.

Philosophical Concerns with CBT Methods

The methods employed in CBT research have not been the only criticisms; some individuals have called its theory and therapy into question. For example, Fancher argues that CBT has failed to provide a framework for clear and correct thinking. He states that it is strange for CBT theorists to develop a framework for determining distorted thinking without ever developing a framework for "cognitive clarity" or what would count as "healthy, normal thinking." Additionally, he writes that irrational thinking cannot be a source of mental and emotional distress when there is no evidence of rational thinking causing psychological well-being. Or, that social psychology has proven the normal cognitive processes of the average person to be irrational, even those who are psychologically well. Fancher also says that the theory of CBT is inconsistent with basic principles and research of rationality, and even ignores many rules of logic. He argues that CBT makes something of thinking that is far less exciting and true than thinking probably is. Among his other arguments are the maintaining of the status quo promoted in CBT, the self-deception encouraged within clients and patients engaged in CBT, how poorly the research is conducted, and some of its basic tenets and norms: "The basic norm of cognitive therapy is this: except for how the patient thinks, everything is ok".

Meanwhile, Slife and Williams write that one of the hidden assumptions in CBT is that of determinism, or the absence of free will. They argue that CBT invokes a type of cause-and-effect relationship with cognition. They state that CBT holds that external stimuli from the environment enter the mind, causing different thoughts that cause emotional states. Nowhere in CBT theory is agency, or free will, accounted for. At its most basic foundational assumptions, CBT holds that human beings have no free will and are just determined by the cognitive processes invoked by external stimuli.

Another criticism of CBT theory, especially as applied to Major Depressive Disorder (MDD), is that it confounds the symptoms of the disorder with its causes.

Side Effects

CBT is generally seen as having very low if any side effects. Calls have been made for more appraisal of CBT side effects.

Society and Culture

The UK's National Health Service announced in 2008 that more therapists would be trained to provide CBT at government expense as part of an initiative called Improving Access to Psychological Therapies (IAPT). NICE said that CBT would become the mainstay of treatment for non-severe depression, with medication used only in cases where CBT had failed. Therapists complained that the data does not fully support the attention and funding CBT receives. Psychotherapist and professor Andrew Samuels stated that this constitutes "a coup, a power play by a community that has suddenly found itself on the brink of corralling an enormous amount of money ... Everyone has been seduced by CBT's apparent cheapness." The UK Council for Psychotherapy issued a press release in 2012 saying that the IAPT's policies were undermining traditional psychotherapy and criticized proposals that would limit some approved therapies to CBT, claiming that they restricted patients to "a watered down version of cognitive behavioural therapy (CBT), often delivered by very lightly trained staff".

NICE also recommends offering CBT to people suffering from schizophrenia, as well as those at risk of suffering from a psychotic episode.

Cognitive Therapy

Cognitive therapy (CT) is a type of psychotherapy developed by American psychiatrist Aaron T. Beck. CT is one of the therapeutic approaches within the larger group of cognitive behavioral therapies (CBT) and was first expounded by Beck in the 1960s. Cognitive therapy is based on the cognitive model, which states that thoughts, feelings and behavior are all connected, and that individuals can move toward overcoming difficulties and meeting their goals by identifying and changing unhelpful or inaccurate thinking, problematic behavior, and distressing emotional responses. This involves the individual working collaboratively with the therapist to develop skills for testing and modifying beliefs, identifying distorted thinking, relating to others in different ways, and changing behaviors. A tailored cognitive case conceptualization is developed by the cognitive therapist as a roadmap to understand the individual's internal reality, select appropriate interventions and identify areas of distress.

History

Becoming disillusioned with long-term psychodynamic approaches based on gaining insight into unconscious emotions and drives, Beck came to the conclusion that the way in which his clients perceived, interpreted and attributed meaning in their daily lives—a process scientifically known as cognition—was a key to therapy. Albert Ellis had been working on similar ideas since the 1950s (Ellis,1956). He called his approach Rational Therapy (RT) at first, then Rational Emotive Therapy (RET) and later Rational Emotive Behavior Therapy (REBT).

Beck outlined his approach in *Depression: Causes and Treatment* in 1967. He later expanded his focus to include anxiety disorders, in *Cognitive Therapy and the Emotional Disorders* in 1976, and other disorders and problems. He also introduced a focus on the underlying "schema"—the fundamental underlying ways in which people process information—about the self, the world or the future.

The new cognitive approach came into conflict with the behaviorism ascendant at the time, which denied that talk of mental causes was scientific or meaningful, rather than simply assessing stimuli and behavioral responses. However, the 1970s saw a general "cognitive revolution" in psychology. Behavioral modification techniques and cognitive therapy techniques became joined together, giving rise to cognitive behavioral therapy. Although cognitive therapy has always included some behavioral components, advocates of Beck's particular approach seek to maintain and establish its integrity as a distinct, clearly standardized form of cognitive behavioral therapy in which the cognitive shift is the key mechanism of change.

Precursors of certain fundamental aspects of cognitive therapy have been identified in various ancient philosophical traditions, particularly Stoicism. For example, Beck's original treatment manual for depression states, "The philosophical origins of cognitive therapy can be traced back to the Stoic philosophers".

As cognitive therapy continued to grow in popularity, the Academy of Cognitive Therapy, a non-profit organization, was created to accredit cognitive therapists, create a forum for members to share emerging research and interventions, and to educate consumer regarding cognitive therapy and related mental health issues.

Basis

Therapy may consist of testing the assumptions which one makes and looking for new information that could help shift the assumptions in a way that leads to different emotional or behavioral reactions. Change may begin by targeting thoughts (to change emotion and behavior), behavior (to change feelings and thoughts), or the individual's goals (by identifying thoughts, feelings or behavior that conflict with the goals). Beck initially focused on depression and developed a list of "errors" (cognitive distortion) in thinking that he proposed could maintain depression, including arbitrary inference, selective abstraction, over-generalization, and magnification (of negatives) and minimization (of positives).

As an example of how CT might work: Having made a mistake at work, a man may believe, "I'm useless and can't do anything right at work." He may then focus on the mistake (which he takes as evidence that his belief is true), and his thoughts about being "useless" are likely to lead to negative emotion (frustration, sadness, hopelessness). Given these thoughts and feelings, he may then begin to avoid challenges at work, which is behavior that could provide even more evidence for him that his belief is true. As a result, any adaptive response and further constructive consequences become unlikely, and he may focus even more on any mistakes he may make, which serve to reinforce the original belief of being "useless." In therapy, this example could be identified as a self-fulfilling prophecy or "problem cycle," and the efforts of the therapist and client would be directed at working together to explore and shift this cycle.

People who are working with a cognitive therapist often practice the use of more flexible ways to think and respond, learning to ask themselves whether their thoughts are completely true, and whether those thoughts are helping them to meet their goals. Thoughts that do not meet this description may then be shifted to something more accurate or helpful, leading to more positive emotion, more desirable behavior, and movement toward the person's goals. Cognitive therapy takes a skill-building approach, where the therapist helps the person to learn and practice these skills independently, eventually "becoming his or her own therapist."

Cognitive Model

The cognitive model was originally constructed following research studies conducted by Aaron Beck to explain the psychological processes in depression. It divides the mind beliefs in three levels:

- Automatic thought
- Intermediate belief
- Core belief or basic belief

In 2014, an update of the cognitive model was proposed, called the Generic Cognitive Model (GCM). The GCM is an update of Beck's model that proposes that psychiatric disorders can be differentiated by the nature of their dysfunctional beliefs. The GCM includes a conceptual framework and a clinical approach for understanding common cognitive processes of mental disorders while specifying the unique features of the specific disorders.

Consistent with the cognitive theory of psychopathology, CT is designed to be structured, directive, active, and time-limited, with the express purpose of identifying, reality-testing, and correcting distorted cognition and underlying dysfunctional beliefs.

Cognitive Restructuring (Methods)

- Activity monitoring and activity scheduling

- Behavioral experiments

- Catching, checking, and changing thoughts

- Collaborative empiricism: therapist and client become investigators by examining the evidence to support or reject the patient's cognitions. Empirical evidence is used to determine whether particular cognitions serve any useful purpose.

- Downward Arrow Technique

- Exposure and response prevention

- Guided discovery: therapist elucidates behavioral problems and faulty thinking by designing new experiences that lead to acquisition of new skills and perspectives. Through both cognitive and behavioral methods, the patient discovers more adaptive ways of thinking and coping with environmental stressors by correcting cognitive processing.

- Mastery and pleasure technique

- Problem solving

- Socratic questioning: involves the creation of a series of questions to a) clarify and define problems, b) assist in the identification of thoughts, images and assumptions, c) examine the meanings of events for the patient, and d) assess the consequences of maintaining maladaptive thoughts and behaviors.

Types

Cognitive therapy

based on the cognitive model, stating that thoughts, feelings and behavior are mutually influenced by each other. Shifting cognition is seen as the main mechanism by which lasting emotional and behavioral changes take place. Treatment is very collaborative, tailored, skill-focused, and based on a case conceptualization.

Rational emotive behavior therapy (REBT)

based on the belief that most problems originate in irrational thought. For instance, perfectionists and pessimists usually suffer from issues related to irrational thinking; for example, if a perfectionist encounters a small failure, he or she might perceive it as a much bigger failure. It is better to establish a reasonable standard emotionally, so the individual can live a balanced life. This form of cognitive therapy is an opportunity for the patient to learn of his current distortions and successfully eliminate them.

Cognitive behavioral therapy (CBT)

a system of approaches drawing from both the cognitive and behavioral systems of psychotherapy.

Unlike Psychodynamic approaches, CBT is transparent to the individual receiving services. At the end of the therapy, an individual will often have learned the cognitive therapy skills well enough to "be their own therapist," decreasing dependence on a therapist to provide the answers.

Application

Depression

According to Beck's theory of the etiology of depression, depressed people acquire a negative schema of the world in childhood and adolescence; children and adolescents who experience depression acquire this negative schema earlier. Depressed people acquire such schemas through a loss of a parent, rejection by peers, bullying, criticism from teachers or parents, the depressive attitude of a parent and other negative events. When the person with such schemas encounters a situation that resembles the original conditions of the learned schema in some way, the negative schemas of the person are activated.

Beck's negative triad holds that depressed people have negative thoughts about themselves, their experiences in the world, and the future. For instance, a depressed person might think, "I didn't get the job because I'm terrible at interviews. Interviewers never like me, and no one will ever want to hire me." In the same situation, a person who is not depressed might think, "The interviewer wasn't paying much attention to me. Maybe she already had someone else in mind for the job. Next time I'll have better luck, and I'll get a job soon." Beck also identified a number of other cognitive distortions, which can contribute to depression, including the following: arbitrary inference, selective abstraction, overgeneralization, magnification and minimization.

In 2008 Beck proposed an integrative developmental model of depression that aims to incorporate research in genetics and neuroscience of depression. This model was updated in 2016 to incorporate multiple levels of analyses, new research, and key concepts (e.g., resilience) within the framework of an evolutionary perspective.

Other Applications

Cognitive therapy has been applied to a very wide range of behavioral health issues including:

- Academic achievement

- Addiction

- Anxiety disorders

- Bipolar disorder

- Low self-esteem

- Phobia

- Schizophrenia

- Substance abuse

- Suicidal ideation

- Weight loss

Criticisms

A criticism has been that clinical studies of CBT efficacy (or any psychotherapy) are not double-blind (i.e., neither subjects nor therapists in psychotherapy studies are blind to the type of treatment). They may be single-blinded, the rater may not know the treatment the patient received, but neither the patients nor the therapists are blinded to the type of therapy given (two out of three of the persons involved in the trial, i.e., all of the persons involved in the treatment, are unblinded). The patient is an active participant in correcting negative distorted thoughts, thus quite aware of the treatment group they are in.

Cognitive Restructuring

Cognitive restructuring (CR) is a psychotherapeutic process of learning to identify and dispute irrational or maladaptive thoughts known as cognitive distortions, such as all-or-nothing thinking (splitting), magical thinking, over-generalization, magnification, and emotional reasoning, which are commonly associated with many mental health disorders. CR employs many strategies, such as Socratic questioning, thought recording, and guided imagery, and is used in many types of therapies, including cognitive behavioral therapy (CBT) and rational emotive behaviour therapy (REBT). A number of studies demonstrate considerable efficacy in using CR-based therapies.

Overview

Cognitive restructuring involves four steps:

1. Identification of problematic cognitions known as "automatic thoughts" (ATs) which are dysfunctional or negative views of the self, world, or future based upon already existing beliefs about oneself, the world, or the future

2. Identification of the cognitive distortions in the ATs

3. Rational disputation of ATs with the Socratic method

4. Development of a rational rebuttal to the ATs

There are six types of automatic thoughts:

1. Self-evaluated thoughts

2. Thoughts about the evaluations of others

3. Evaluative thoughts about the other person with whom they are interacting

4. Thoughts about coping strategies and behavioral plans

5. Thoughts of avoidance

6. Any other thoughts that were not categorized

Clinical Applications

Cognitive restructuring has been used to help individuals experiencing a variety of psychiatric conditions, including depression, substance abuse disorders, anxiety disorders collectively, bulimia, social phobia, borderline personality disorder, attention deficit hyperactivity disorder (ADHD), and problem gambling.

When utilizing cognitive restructuring in rational emotive therapy (RET), the emphasis is on two central notions: (1) thoughts affect human emotion as well as behavior and (2) irrational beliefs are mainly responsible for a wide range of disorders. RET also classifies four types of irrational beliefs: dire necessity, feeling awful, cannot stand something, and self-condemnation. It is described as cognitive-emotional retraining. The rationale used in cognitive restructuring attempts to strengthen the client's belief that (1) "self-talk" can influence performance, and (2) in particular self-defeating thoughts or negative self-statements can cause emotional distress and interfere with performance, a process that then repeats again in a cycle. Mood repair strategies are implemented in cognitive restructuring in hopes of contributing to a cessation of the negative cycle.

When utilizing cognitive restructuring in cognitive behavioral therapy (CBT), it is combined with psychoeducation, monitoring, *in vivo* experience, imaginal exposure, behavioral activation, and homework assignments to achieve remission. The cognitive behavioral approach is said to consist of three core techniques: cognitive restructuring, training in coping skills, and problem solving.

Applications within Therapy

There are many methods used in cognitive restructuring, which usually involve identifying and labelling distorted thoughts, such as "all or none thinking, disqualifying the positive, mental filtering, jumping to conclusions, catastrophizing, emotional reasoning, should statements, and personalization." The following lists methods commonly used in cognitive restructuring:

- Socratic questioning

- Thought recording

- Identifying cognitive errors

- Examining the evidence (pro-con analysis or cost-benefits analysis)

- Understanding idiosyncratic meaning/semantic techniques

- Labeling distortions

- Decatastrophizing

- Reattribution

- Cognitive rehearsal

- Guided imagery

- Listing rational alternatives

Criticism

Critics of cognitive restructuring claim that the process of challenging dysfunctional thoughts will "teach clients to become better suppressors and avoiders of their unwanted thoughts" and that cognitive restructuring shows less immediate improvement because real-world practice is often required. Other criticisms include that the approach is mechanistic and impersonal and that the relationship between therapist and client is irrelevant.

Beck's Cognitive Triad

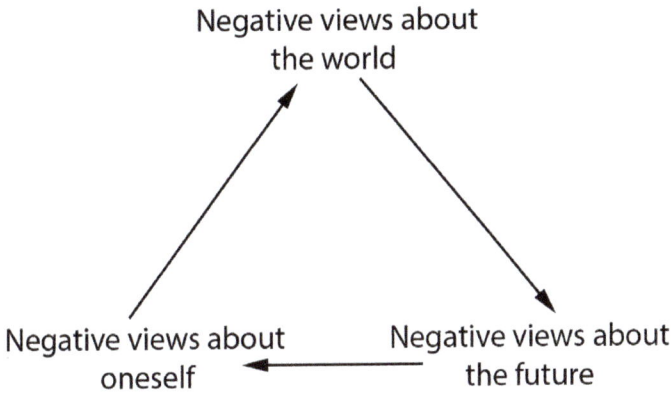

A diagram showing Beck's cognitive triad

Beck's cognitive triad, also known as the negative triad, is an irrational and pessimistic view of the three key elements of a person's belief system present in depression. It was proposed by Aaron Beck in 1976. The triad forms part of his cognitive theory of depression and the concept is used as part of CBT, particularly in Beck's "Treatment of Negative Automatic Thoughts" (TNAT) approach.

The triad involves "automatic, spontaneous and seemingly uncontrollable negative thoughts" about:

- The *self*
- The *world or environment*
- The *future*

Examples of this negative thinking include:

- The self – "I'm worthless and ugly" or "I wish I was different"
- The world – "No one values me" or "people ignore me all the time"
- The future – "I'm hopeless because things will never change" or "things can only get worse!"

Beck's Cognitive Model of Depression

From a cognitive perspective, depressive disorders are characterized by people's dysfunctional negative views of themselves, their life experience (and the world in general), and their future—the cognitive triad.

People with depression often view themselves as unlovable, helpless, doomed or deficient. They tend to attribute their unpleasant experiences to their presumed physical, mental, and/or moral deficits. They tend to feel excessively guilty, believing that they are worthless, blameworthy, and rejected by self and others. They may have a very difficult time viewing themselves as people who could ever succeed, be accepted, or feel good about themselves and this may lead to withdrawal and isolation, which further worsens the mood.

Cognitive Distortions

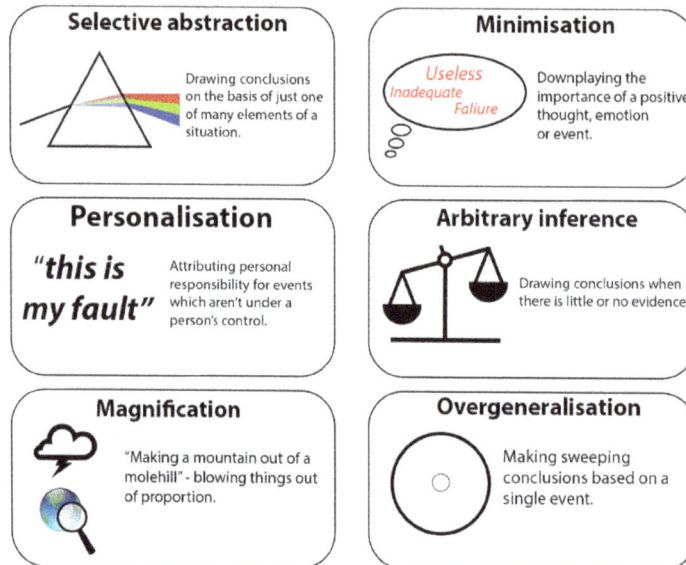

Examples of some of the cognitive biases used by depressed individuals, according to cognitive theories including Beck's cognitive model. People with depression may be taught how to identify and alter these biases as part of Cognitive Behavioural Therapy.

Beck proposes that those with depression develop cognitive distortions, a type of cognitive bias sometimes also referred to as faulty or unhelpful thinking patterns. Beck referred to some of these biases as "automatic thoughts", suggesting they are not entirely under conscious control. People with depression will tend to quickly overlook their positive attributes and disqualify their accomplishments as being minor or meaningless. They may also misinterpret the care, good will, and concern of others as being based on pity or susceptible to being lost easily if those others knew the "real person" and this fuels further feelings of guilt. The main cognitive distortions according to Beck are summarised below:

- Arbitrary inference - drawing conclusions from insufficient or no evidence.

- Selective abstraction - drawing conclusions on the basis on just one of many elements of a situation.

- Overgeneralisation - making sweeping conclusions based on a single event.

- Magnification - exaggerating the importance of an undesirable event.

- Minimisation - underplaying the significance of a positive event.

- Personalisation - attributing negative feelings of others to oneself.

Depressed people view their lives as devoid of pleasure or reward, presenting insuperable obstacles to achieving their important goals. This is often manifested as a lack of motivation and leads to the depressed person feeling further withdrawal and isolation as they may be seen as lazy by others. Everything seems and feels "too hard to manage" and other people are seen as punishing (or potentially so). They believe that their troubles will continue indefinitely, and that the future will only bring further hardship, deprivation, and frustration. "Paralysis of the will" results from the depressed patients' pessimism and hopelessness. Expecting their efforts to end in failure, they are reluctant to commit themselves to growth-oriented goals, and their activity level drops. Believing that they cannot affect the outcome of various situations, they experience a desire to avoid such situations.

Suicidal wishes are seen as an extreme expression of the desire to escape from problems that appear to be uncontrollable, interminable, and unbearable.

Negative self-schemata

Beck also believed that a depressed person will, often from childhood experiences, hold a negative self-schema. This schema may originate from negative early experiences, such as criticism, abuse or bullying. Beck suggests that people with negative self-schemata are liable to interpret information presented to them in a negative manner, leading to the cognitive distortions outlined above. The pessimistic explanatory style, which describes the way in which depressed or neurotic people react negatively to certain events, is an example of the effect of these schemata on self-image. This explanatory style involves blaming oneself for negative events outside of their control or the behaviour of others (personalisation), believing that such events will continue forever and letting these events significantly affect their emotional wellbeing.

Measuring Aspects of the Triad

A number of instruments have been developed to attempt to measure negative cognition in the three areas of the triad. The Beck Depression Inventory (BDI) is a well-known questionnaire for scoring depression based on all three aspects of the triad. Other examples include the Beck Hopelessness Scale for measuring thoughts about the future and the Rosenberg Self-Esteem Scale for measuring views of the self. The Cognitive Triad Inventory (CTI) was developed by Beckham *et al.* to attempt to systematically measure the three aspects of Beck's triad. The CTI aims to quantify the relationship between "therapist behaviour in a single treatment session to changes in the cognitive triad" and "patterns of changes to the triad to changes in overall depressive mood". This inventory has since been adapted for use with children and adolescents in the CTI-C, developed by Kaslow *et al.*

Cognitive Distortion

Cognitive distortions are exaggerated or irrational thought patterns that are believed to perpetuate the effects of psychopathological states, especially depression and anxiety. Psychiatrist Aaron T. Beck laid the groundwork for the study of these distortions, and his student David D. Burns continued research on the topic. Burns's *The Feeling Good Handbook* (1989) describes these thought patterns and how to eliminate them.

Cognitive distortions are thoughts that cognitive therapists believe cause individuals to perceive reality inaccurately. These thinking patterns often are said to reinforce negative thoughts or emotions. Cognitive distortions tend to interfere with the way a person perceives an event. Because the way a person feels intervenes with how they think, these distorted thoughts can feed negative emotions and lead an individual affected by cognitive distortions towards an overall negative outlook on the world and consequently a depressive or anxious mental state.

History

In 1972, psychiatrist, psychoanalyst, and cognitive therapy scholar Aaron T. Beck published *Depression: Causes and Treatment*. Dissatisfied with the conventional Freudian treatment of depression, he concluded that there was no empirical evidence for the success of Freudian psychoanalysis in the understanding or treatment of depression. In his book, Beck provided a comprehensive and empirically supported look at depression — its potential causes, symptoms, and treatments. In Chapter 2, "Symptomatology of Depression," he describes certain "cognitive manifestations" of depression, including low self-evaluation, negative expectations, self-blame and self-criticism, indecisiveness, and distortion of body image.

In 1980 Burns published *Feeling Good: The New Mood Therapy* (with a preface from Beck), and nine years later published *The Feeling Good Handbook*. These books built on Beck's work, delving deeper into the definition, development, and treatment of cognitive distortions, specifically in regards to depression or anxiety disorders.

Main Types

The cognitive distortions listed below are categories of automatic thinking, and are to be distinguished from logical fallacies.

Always Being Right

Being wrong is unthinkable. This cognitive distortion is characterized by actively trying to prove one's actions or thoughts to be correct, while sometimes prioritizing self-interest over the feelings of another person.

Blaming

The opposite of *personalization*; holding other people responsible for the harm they cause, and especially for their intentional or negligent infliction of emotional distress.

> Example: someone blames their spouse entirely for marital problems, instead of looking at his/her own part in the problems.

Disqualifying the Positive

Discounting positive events.

- Example: Upon receiving a congratulation, a person dismisses it out-of-hand, believing it to be undeserved, and automatically interpreting the compliment (at least inwardly) as an attempt at flattery or perhaps as arising out of naïveté.

Emotional Reasoning

Presuming that negative feelings expose the true nature of things, and experiencing reality as a reflection of emotionally linked thoughts. Thinking something is true, solely based on a feeling.

- Example: "I feel (i.e. think that I am) stupid or boring, therefore I must be." Or, feeling that fear of flying in planes means planes are a very dangerous way to travel. Or, concluding that it's hopeless to clean one's house due to being overwhelmed by the prospect of cleaning.

Fallacy of Change

Relying on social control to obtain cooperative actions from another person.

Fallacy of Fairness

Becoming guilty when one acts against justice or upset when someone else acts unjustly.

Filtering

Focusing entirely on negative elements of a situation, to the exclusion of the positive. Also, the brain's tendency to filter out information which does not conform to already held beliefs.

- Example: After receiving comments about a work presentation, a person focuses on the single critical comment and ignores what went well.

Jumping to Conclusions

Reaching preliminary conclusions (usually negative) from little (if any) evidence. Two specific subtypes are identified:

- Mind reading: Inferring a person's possible or probable (usually negative) thoughts from their behavior and nonverbal communication; taking precautions against the worst reasonably suspected case or some other preliminary conclusion, without asking the person.

    o Example: A student assumes the readers of their paper have already made up their mind concerning its topic, and therefore writing the paper is a pointless exercise.

- Fortune-telling: predicting outcomes (usually negative) of events.

    o Example: Being convinced of failure before a test, when the student is in fact prepared.

Labeling and Mislabeling

A more severe type of overgeneralization; attributing a person's actions to their character instead of some accidental attribute. Rather than assuming the behavior to be accidental or extrinsic, the person assigns a label to someone or something that implies the character of that person or thing. Mislabeling involves describing an event with language that has a strong connotation of a person's evaluation of the event.

- Example of "labeling": Instead of believing that you made a mistake, you believe that you are a loser, because only a loser would make that kind of mistake. Or, someone who made a bad first impression is a "jerk", in the absence of some more specific cause.

- Example of "mislabeling": A woman who places her children in a day care center is "abandoning her children to strangers," because the person who says so highly values the bond between mother and child.

Magnification and Minimization

Giving proportionally greater weight to a perceived failure, weakness or threat, or lesser weight to a perceived success, strength or opportunity, so the weight differs from that assigned to the event or thing by others. This is common enough in the normal population to popularize idioms such as "make a mountain out of a molehill". In depressed clients, often the positive characteristics of *other people* are exaggerated and negative characteristics are understated. There is one subtype of magnification:

- Catastrophizing – Giving greater weight to the worst possible outcome, however unlikely, or experiencing a situation as unbearable or impossible when it is just uncomfortable.

- Example: A teenager is too afraid to start driver's training because he believes he would get himself into an accident.

Overgeneralization

Making hasty generalizations from insufficient experiences and evidence. Making a very broad conclusion based on a single incident or a single piece of evidence. If something bad happens only once, it is expected to happen over and over again.

- Example: A person is lonely and often spends most of her time at home. Her friends sometimes ask her to come out for dinner and meet new people. She feels it is useless to try to meet people. No one really could like her.

Personalization

Attributing personal responsibility, including the resulting praise or blame, for events over which a person has no control.

- Example: A mother whose child is struggling in school blames herself entirely for being a bad mother, because she believes that her deficient parenting is responsible. In fact, the real cause may be something else entirely.

Should Statements

Doing, or expecting others to do, what they morally should or ought to do irrespective of the particular case the person is faced with. This involves conforming strenuously to ethical categorical imperatives which, by definition, "always apply," or to hypothetical imperatives which apply in that general type of case. Albert Ellis termed this "musturbation". Psychotherapist Michael C. Graham describes this as "expecting the world to be different than it is".

- Example: After a performance, a concert pianist believes he or she should not have made so many mistakes.

- David Burns' *Feeling Good: The New Mood Therapy* does not distinguish between pathological "should statements," moral imperatives, and social norms.

Splitting (All-or-nothing thinking or dichotomous reasoning)

Evaluating the self, as well as events in life in extreme terms. It's either all good or all bad, either black or white, nothing in between. Causing every small imperfection to seem incredibly dangerous and painful. Splitting involves using terms like "always", "every" or "never" when this is neither true nor equivalent to the truth.

- Example: When an admired person makes a minor mistake, the admiration is turned into contempt.

Cognitive Restructuring

Cognitive restructuring (CR) is a popular form of therapy used to identify and break down maladaptive cognitive distortions. It is typically used with individuals with depression. CR therapies aim to eliminate "automatic thoughts" which create dysfunctional or negative views for individuals. Cognitive restructuring is the main component of Beck's and Burns's cognitive behavioral therapy (CBT).

As Narcissistic Defense

Exaggeration and minimization are commonly adopted by narcissists to manage and defend against psychic pain.

Decatastrophizing

In cognitive therapy, decatastrophizing or decatastrophization is a cognitive restructuring technique to treat cognitive distortions, such as magnification and catastrophizing, commonly seen in psychological disorders like anxiety and psychosis.

References

- Elkins, Gary; Johnson, Aimee; Fisher, William (2012). "Cognitive Hypnotherapy for Pain Management". American Journal of Clinical Hypnosis. 54 (4): 294–310. PMID 22655332. doi:10.1080/00029157.2011.654284

- Hofmann SG (2011). An Introduction to Modern CBT. Psychological Solutions to Mental Health Problems. Chichester, UK: Wiley-Blackwell. ISBN 0-470-97175-4

- "Depression and anxiety – computerised cognitive behavioural therapy (CCBT)". National Institute for Health and Care Excellence. 2012-01-12. Retrieved 2012-02-04

- O'Brian, S.; Onslow, M. (2011). "Clinical management of stuttering in children and adults". BMJ. 342: d3742. PMID 21705407. doi:10.1136/bmj.d3742

- Hoffman, Stefan G.; Smits, Jasper A. J. (2008). "Cognitive-Behavioral Therapy for Adult Anxiety Disorders". The Journal of Clinical Psychiatry. 69 (4): 621–32. PMC 2409267. PMID 18363421. doi:10.4088/JCP.v69n0415

- Reinicke, M., Dattillo, F., Freeman, A., (Eds.), 2003. Cognitive Therapy with Children and Adolescents, Second Edition: A Casebook for Clinical Practice. ISBN 978-1572308534

- "A Step By Step Guide to Delivering Guided Self Help CBT" (PDF). Archived from the original (PDF) on October 24, 2012. Retrieved April 9, 2013

- Gardenswartz, Cara Ann; Craske, Michelle G. (2001). "Prevention of panic disorder". Behavior Therapy. 32 (4): 725–37. doi:10.1016/S0005-7894(01)80017-4

- Wilson G.D. (1968). "Reversal of differential conditioning by instructions". Journal of Experimental Psychology. 76: 491–493. doi:10.1037/h0025540

- Donald Robertson (2010). The Philosophy of Cognitive-Behavioural Therapy: Stoicism as Rational and Cognitive Psychotherapy. London: Karnac. p. xix. ISBN 978-1-85575-756-1

- Laurance J (December 16, 2008). "The big question: can cognitive behavioural therapy help people with eating disorders?". The Independent. Retrieved April 22, 2012

- Huppert J.D. (2009). "The building blocks of treatment in cognitive-behavioral therapy". Israel Journal of Psychiatry Related Science. 46: 245–250

- Hofmann SG (2011). An Introduction to Modern CBT: Psychological Solutions to Mental Health Problems. Wiley-Blackwell. p. 236. ISBN 0-470-97175-4

- Goode, Erica (11 January 2000). "A Pragmatic Man and His No-Nonsense Therapy". The New York Times. Retrieved 2008-11-21

- Williams, C. (2001). "Use of written cognitive-behavioural therapy self-help materials to treat depression". Advances in Psychiatric Treatment. 7 (3): 233–40. doi:10.1192/apt.7.3.233

- Joseph, J.S.; Gray, M.J. (2008). "Exposure Therapy for Posttraumatic Stress Disorder". Journal of Behavior Analysis of Offender and Victim: Treatment and Prevention. 1 (4): 69–80. doi:10.1037/h0100457

- Sadock, Sadock, Ruiz, Benjamin J., Virginia Alcott, Pedro (2009). Kaplan and Sadock's Comprehensive Textbook of Psychiatry. Lippincott Williams and Wilkins. ISBN 9780781768993

- C. Becker; C. Zayfert; E. Anderson. "A Survey of Psychologists' Attitudes Towards and Utilization of Exposure Therapy for PTSD". Digital Commons @ Trinity. Retrieved 13 June 2011

- Lincoln, TM (2010). "Letter to the editor: A comment on Lynch et al. (2009)". Psychological Medicine. 40 (5): 877–80. PMID 19917145. doi:10.1017/S0033291709991838

CPSIA information can be obtained
at www.ICGtesting.com
Printed in the USA
LVHW020136050719
623148LV00004B/40/P

9 781632 425577